Fundamentals of
Neuroimaging

Fundamentals of Neuroimaging

Blaine L. Hart, MD

Associate Professor of Radiology
Department of Radiology
University of New Mexico
Health Sciences Center
School of Medicine
Albuquerque, New Mexico

Edward C. Benzel, MD

Professor and Chief of Neurosurgery
University of New Mexico
Health Sciences Center
School of Medicine
Albuquerque, New Mexico

Corey C. Ford, MD

Associate Professor of Neurology
Department of Neurology
University of New Mexico
Health Sciences Center
School of Medicine
Albuquerque, New Mexico

W.B. SAUNDERS COMPANY
A Division of Harcourt Brace & Company
Philadelphia London Toronto Montreal Sydney Tokyo

W.B. SAUNDERS COMPANY
A Division of Harcourt Brace & Company

The Curtis Center
Independence Square West
Philadelphia, Pennsylvania 19106

Library of Congress Cataloging-in-Publication Data

Hart, Blaine L.

Fundamentals of neuroimaging / Blaine L. Hart, Edward C. Benzel,
Corey C. Ford.—1st ed.

p.   cm.

ISBN 0–7216–5163–1

1. Brain—Imaging.   2. Spinal cord—Imaging.   I. Benzel, Edward C.
II. Ford, Corey C.   III. Title.
[DNLM: 1. Neuroradiography—methods.   2. Brain Diseases—radiography.
3. Diagnostic Imaging—methods.   4. Spinal Diseases—radiography.
WL 141 H325f 1997]

RC386.6.D52H37 1997   616.8′04754—dc20

DNLM/DLC   96-7421

FUNDAMENTALS OF NEUROIMAGING   ISBN 0–7216–5163–1

Printed in the United States of America.

Last digit is the print number: 9   8   7   6   5   4   3   2   1

To Nancy
BLH

To Mary
ECB

To Chad
CCF

Preface

The purpose of this book is to provide an introduction to neuroimaging in clinical practice. By combining the viewpoints of a neuroradiologist, neurosurgeon, and neurologist, we have sought to provide an anatomic and a clinical perspective along with insight into common diagnostic challenges.

For the most part, we have concentrated on principles of imaging studies and characteristics of common disorders of the central nervous system. A few uncommon entities have been illustrated because they are clinically important or distinctive or demonstrate important concepts. It is our hope that the clinician who has had limited experience with neuroimaging and the beginning resident will find this book a useful overview. Because of the limitations of size and scope, details are necessarily limited; we recommend to interested readers the many other excellent texts and learning resources now available on neuroimaging.

An introductory discussion on an approach to imaging of the brain is followed by chapters on trauma, infection, tumors, and vascular diseases of the brain. The imaging of hydrocephalus, a condition that may arise from a variety of etiologies, is also presented. We have emphasized multiple sclerosis within the context of neurodegenerative disorders, along with a survey of other related disease processes. Neurologic conditions distinctive to children complete the section on imaging of the brain. The discussion of spinal imaging includes fundamental principles, congenital disorders, spinal trauma, and acquired disorders such as degenerative, infectious, neoplastic, and vascular diseases.

We look forward to the day when technology for remote viewing of images is universally available. Until that time, however, verbal communication regarding CT images is often necessary between a physician who has access to the scan and another who does not. The images in Appendix 1 are provided as an elementary aid to the objective and quantitative description of the size of subdural and epidural hematomas. Appendix 2 provides a simplified initial guide to the imaging of common CNS disorders.

We acknowledge the contributions of our colleagues in providing cases or material for this book. We thank Frederick W. Rupp, M.D., Fred A. Mettler, Jr., M.D., and Cary Alberstone, M.D., for their review of the manuscript and suggestions, and Gabriela Miranda and Floyd Willard for their editorial and photographic expertise.

Blaine L. Hart
Edward C. Benzel
Corey C. Ford

Contents

1. Imaging Techniques and Brain Anatomy 1

2. Cranial Trauma 11

3. Infections of the Brain and Meninges 25

4. Neoplasms of the Brain 39

5. Ischemia and Related Vascular Diseases of the Brain 67

6. Intracranial Hemorrhage and Related
   Vascular Diseases 79

7. Hydrocephalus 95

8. Multiple Sclerosis and Degenerative
   Diseases of the Brain 103

9. Pediatric Neuroradiology 111

10. Approach to Imaging the Spine: Anatomy,
    Development, and Disorders of Development 135

11. Spinal Trauma 145

12. Nontraumatic Acquired Disorders of the Spine 161

Further Readings 183

Appendix 1 185

Appendix 2 189

Index 191

1

Imaging Techniques and Brain Anatomy

Cross-sectional imaging techniques—computed tomography (CT) and magnetic resonance imaging (MRI)—are currently the most widely used clinical tools for imaging the brain. They are readily available and involve relatively limited risks. Myelography and angiography, which were used much more frequently in the past, are still useful for specific applications despite their more invasive nature. Ultrasound testing has more limited utility for the central nervous system (CNS) than elsewhere in the body because of the limitations created by encasing bone. Ultrasound testing is, however, especially helpful for pediatric and intraoperative applications. Nuclear medicine tests have poor spatial resolution. However, occasionally there are compensating advantages related to the physiologic foundation of the study. Various advanced imaging techniques are employed for research purposes that may prove to be clinically efficacious.

In this chapter, a brief discussion of basic brain anatomy, as visualized by cross-sectional imaging, is followed by an overview of fundamental principles of CNS imaging techniques. Standard convention for axial CT and MRI, used throughout this book, is to film the images as if looking through a cross-section from the foot of the patient's bed. Thus, the *patient's right side* is on the *left side of the image*.

BASIC BRAIN ANATOMY ON CROSS-SECTIONAL IMAGING

In evaluating CT or MRI scans, as with any imaging study, it is important to have a systematic approach. An orderly and consistent method of analyzing scans ensures that all major features are inspected, and that obvious abnormalities do not distract attention from more subtle lesions. Complete evaluation includes consideration of the ventricular system; the extra-axial cerebrospinal fluid (CSF) spaces; the brain itself; blood vessels when possible; visualized portions of the skull; and visualized portions of the paranasal sinuses, orbits, and extracranial soft tissues. Foreign bodies, limiting technical features, or artifacts should also be noted.

Abnormalities can be characterized in several ways: altered attenuation (on CT) or signal intensity (on MRI), anatomic location, and evidence of either mass effect or volume loss (see Fig. 5–3). Categorizing an intracranial mass as intra-axial (within the brain) or extra-axial (outside the brain) is the first step in the localization process; differential diagnoses vary for these two types of diseases. Location can be further described according to the region of the brain involved.

The ventricles contain about 40 ml of CSF. The total volume of CSF, which includes CSF around the brain and spine as well as within the ventricles, is about 120 to 150 ml. These volumes, however, may vary significantly.

Some asymmetry of the bodies and frontal horns of the lateral ventricles is common. The third and fourth ventricles should lie in the midline. The size of normal cortical sulci and amount of CSF visible over the convexities of the brain vary with age. Some degree of age-related diffuse volume loss is inevitable. The CSF cisterns around the brainstem and base of the brain should be inspected when evaluating appropriate imaging studies. They include the prepontine; cerebellopontine angle (CPA); quadrigeminal plate; and ambient and suprasellar cisterns. Effacement of these cisterns often provides important clues regarding edema and mass effect.

The major divisions of the brain (the lobes, deep gray matter nuclei and internal capsule, midbrain, pons, and medulla) may be demonstrated by CT and MRI. A high degree of right-left symmetry is present normally, although subtle but distinct differences can be found that are related to cerebral dominance.

A mini-atlas of CT and MR images of the brain at representative levels is portrayed in Figure 1–1. Numerous atlases are available for more detailed reference.

COMPUTED TOMOGRAPHY

Physical Basis of CT

Computed tomography (CT) was the first cross-sectional imaging test available for the brain, and it remains the test of choice for many clinical situations. *Tomography* is a term that refers to a method of producing images of a plane. With CT, a rotating x-ray beam and detectors located circumferentially around the body send information from the detectors to a computer, and a computerized back-projection technique reconstructs a two-dimensional image based on the attenuation characteristics. As with conventional x-ray techniques (plain radiography), bone and other dense objects appear bright, and less dense material appears darker. From a practical standpoint, it is important to note that bone can be visualized well with CT. CT, however, is prone to the generation of artifact at bone/soft tissue interfaces. For example, the posterior fossa between the petrous portions of the temporal bones is often the site of CT artifact, limiting visualization of the brainstem.

Tissue Characteristics on CT

CT discrimination of different soft tissue structures is far superior to that of conventional radiographs. Air and fat characteristically have low attenuation and are readily identified. CSF is very similar in attenuation to water. Gray and white matter are denser than CSF and are normally different enough from each other to be distinguished. Flowing (normal) blood is denser than brain, and acute hematoma is denser still due to clot retraction and loss of water.

Pathologic processes in the brain are often detected by CT because of the presence of surrounding edema, which is less dense than normal brain. However, increased density within the lesion can occur with some conditions, especially tumors with a high nuclear-to-cytoplasmic ratio. Calcification is also readily detected by CT. The use of intravenously injected, iodinated contrast medium leads to enhancement (high density) in two situations: (1) increased vascularity and (2) breakdown of the blood-brain barrier.

Safety Considerations with CT

CT has very little risk. Radiation is limited because the beam is very tightly collimated. Furthermore, the standard plane for CT imaging of the brain is deliberately selected to avoid excessive radiation to the lens of the eye. Patient motion causes artifact, and thus sedation is occasionally necessary. CT images are acquired very quickly (with current equipment, usually a few seconds for one slice and a matter of minutes for an entire examination). Because intravenous contrast material administration always entails a small risk of adverse reaction, its use must be carefully considered, especially with the ready availability of MRI.

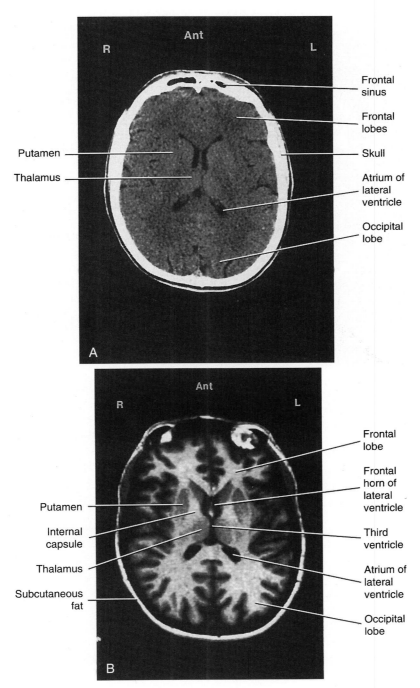

Figure 1–1. Normal brain anatomy on cross-sectional imaging. *(A)* Axial CT through the level of the internal capsule and basal ganglia. *(B)* Axial MRI, T1-weighted image (T1WI), through the level of the internal capsule and basal ganglia.

Illustration continued on following page

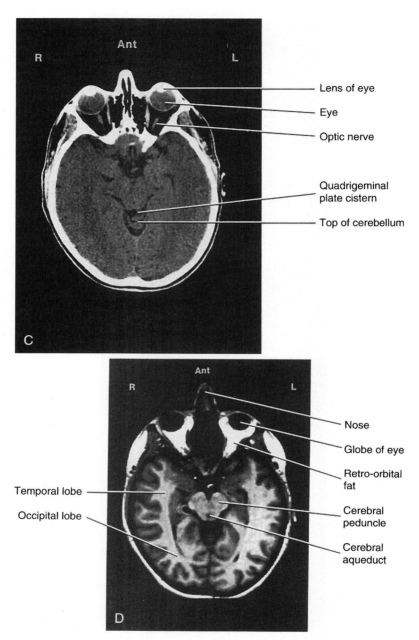

Figure 1–1 *Continued (C)* Axial CT through the level of the midbrain. *(D)* Axial MRI (T1WI) through the level of the midbrain.

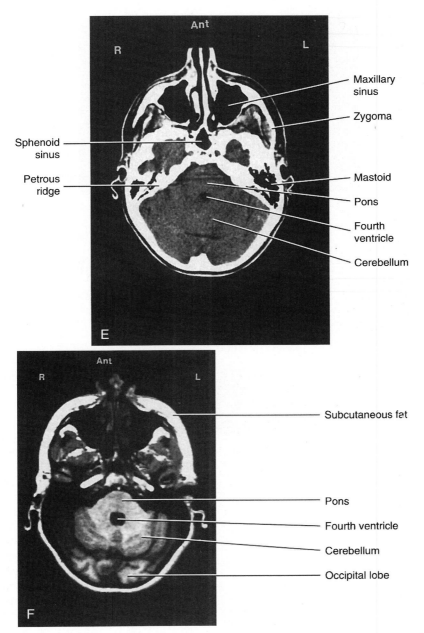

Figure 1–1 *Continued (E)* Axial CT through the level of the fourth ventricle and pons. *(F)* Axial MRI (T1WI) through the level of the fourth ventricle and pons.

Illustration continued on following page

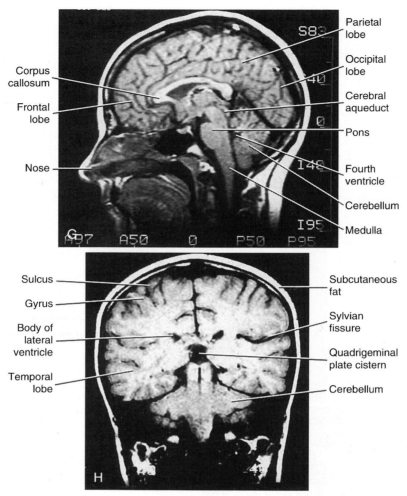

Figure 1–1 *Continued (G)* Sagittal MRI (T1WI), midline. *(H)* Coronal MRI (T1WI) through the level of the brainstem. (From Mettler F: Essentials of Radiology. Philadelphia, WB Saunders, 1995, pp 19–22.)

MAGNETIC RESONANCE IMAGING

Physical Basis of MRI

Magnetic resonance imaging (MRI) produces cross-sectional images that bear some similarity to those of CT, but the physical foundation is completely different. Magnetic resonance images are based on signals derived from the protons associated with tissue water and, to a lesser extent, fat. The physical principle underlying MRI is the weak magnetic property of the hydrogen proton. Within a very strong magnetic field, there is a tendency for spinning hydrogen protons to align with the external magnetic field. When a brief radiofrequency (RF) pulse is applied with a frequency matching that of the hydrogen protons (magnetic resonance), the net magnetization direction of the protons is altered, and the protons are transiently in phase. An extremely weak electronic signal is generated by the perturbed protons. As soon as the external electronic pulse stops, the signal begins to disappear. The signal loss is the result of two independent factors: (1) the protons begin to return to alignment with the static, external magnetic field (spin-lattice relaxation); and (2) interactions between nearby molecules disrupt phase coherence (spin-spin relaxation). Both processes evolve by exponential decay kinetics. The mathematic description of these processes is expressed using a time constant, which is T1 for spin-lattice relaxation and T2 for spin-spin relaxation.

Converting the Signal from Protons into Images

Highly sensitive equipment is necessary to detect the weak (and rapidly decaying) signals arising from the protons. Although a large coil within the bore of an MRI system can serve as an antenna for body imaging applications, the best signal detection is achieved when specialized coils (antennas) are used that are close to the body part imaged. For CNS applications, these include special coils that surround the head and spine coils that are either curved (for the neck) or flat (for the thoracic and lumbar spine).

It is necessary to further modify the process to gain the spatial information necessary to reconstruct an image. Modification typically involves imposing a slight directional gradient on the magnetic field (frequency-encoding) and applying additional pulses to alter phase (phase-encoding). Mathematic techniques, including Fourier transformation of the measured signal, are used to produce an image (representing signal intensity) from each element (volume element or voxel) in a matrix. Unlike CT, MRI is readily acquired in any desired plane. The signal intensity arising from a given location depends on several factors: (1) the T1 and T2 relaxation properties of the tissue; (2) number of protons present (proton density); and (3) gross movement of protons during the acquisition of the image, especially flowing blood or CSF.

How does such esoteric-appearing and complex data acquisition produce meaningful information? The specific method of stimulating tissue with radiofrequency energy and measuring a response—the pulse sequences used—can be tailored to emphasize certain tissue characteristics. Knowledge can be gained not only about anatomy but also about pathologic processes. Some information is tissue-specific, whereas other features of MRI are not specific but are highly sensitive to conditions such as edema.

TE, TR, and More: What Do They Mean?

A brief introduction to terminology may be helpful in understanding discussion and literature about MRI. As mentioned earlier, the electromagnetic signal generated by magnetic resonance decays very quickly. To counter this, most clinical systems use spin-echo (SE) and/or gradient-echo (or gradient-recall, GR) techniques for routine imaging. These cause a reversal of either proton spin or gradient direction to regain a measurable signal (an echo). It is possible to produce multiple echoes, each with less peak intensity, after an initial pulse. In gradient-echo imaging, the RF energy deposited causes a change in net magnetization vector (flip angle) of less than 90 degrees; 90- and 180-degree flip angles are used for most spin-echo imaging. *Flip angle* in degrees, *repetition time (TR)* in milliseconds between pulse sequences, and time in milliseconds from refocusing pulse to the measured echo *(echo time, or TE)* are commonly used terms in MRI.

Spin-echo sequences with short TR and short TE produce images in which the T1 of tissue is a major determinant of signal intensity, and thus they are sometimes referred to as *T1-weighted images* (T1WIs). Long TR and long TE result in images weighted heavily by the T2 of tissue, or *T2-weighted images* (T2WIs). During that same sequence, long TR and short TE images can be obtained by measuring an earlier echo. These images have intermediate characteristics and are occasionally referred to as *proton-density images.* However, they are not truly images of proton density but, like all routine MR images, are influenced by a mixture of T1, T2, and proton density.

Tissue Characteristics on MRI

Fat has a short T1 and appears very bright on T1-weighted images. Fat has lower signal intensity and appears dark on routine long TR/long TE (T2-weighted) images, but it remains bright on fast imaging techniques that use a train of multiple echoes.

The appearance of fat alone, therefore, cannot be relied upon to identify the type of pulse sequence used.

Water has a long T1 and long T2 and appears relatively dark on T1-weighted images and very bright on T2-weighted images. CSF and vitreous humor, for example, should be very bright on long TR/long TE SE images. More importantly, edema, which is present with many pathologic processes in the brain and spine, is also bright. Long TR/short TE, or intermediate-weighted, images are particularly helpful in that CSF is less intense (less bright) than on long TE images, but edema remains bright. Brightness characteristics are especially helpful for detecting abnormalities that lie adjacent to the ventricular system or sulci, where they can be inseparable from bright CSF on long TE images. Normal white matter is brighter than gray matter on T1-weighted images and darker on T2-weighted images. T1-weighted SE images are acquired relatively quickly and yield excellent spatial and anatomic information. T2-weighted images take longer to acquire and have poorer signal-to-noise ratio. However, they are more sensitive to edema and hence to most disease states. Signal characteristics of common tissues and materials are summarized in Table 1–1.

Air and dense bone contain few mobile hydrogen protons and appear black on MRI. This MRI "invisibility" of bone is beneficial in evaluating areas such as the brainstem that are obscured by CT artifact. If alteration of bone is of concern, CT may be necessary.

The MRI appearance of blood is complex and is discussed in further detail in Chapter 6. Calcium usually gives little signal on MRI and appears dark, but in some situations calcium within tissue can appear bright on T1-weighted images. (Calcium is detected more consistently with CT.) Fat and vascular tissue within bone marrow give MR signal. MRI is very sensitive to bone marrow pathology despite its insensitivity to cortical bone changes.

Gradient-echo images also reflect varying degrees of T1 or T2 weighting. These sequences are acquired more quickly than SE sequences. They are more sensitive than SE sequences to factors causing local perturbations of the magnetic field, including hemorrhage.

TABLE 1–1. **MRI Characteristics of Common Structures**

Dark on T1-weighted Sequences

Bone
Air
Flowing blood (spin-echo sequences)
Calcium (dense)

Bright on T1-weighted Sequences

Fat
Methemoglobin
Flowing blood (gradient-echo sequences)
Calcium, some circumstances
Gadolinium-based contrast agents

Brain Tissues on T1-weighted Sequences

White matter brighter than gray matter
Water dark gray, fat bright

Dark on T2-weighted Sequences

Bone
Air
Flowing blood (spin-echo sequences)
Calcium (dense)
Deoxyhemoglobin
Hemosiderin, blood breakdown products
Methemoglobin (intracellular)
Fat
Iron-laden tissues

Bright on T2-weighted Sequences

Methemoglobin (extracellular)
Water
CSF
Flowing blood (gradient-echo sequences)

Brain Tissues on T2-weighted Sequences

Gray matter brighter than white matter
Water very bright, fat dark gray*

*Fat stays bright on fast spin-echo sequences.

MRI Contrast Agents

Several chelates of gadolinium are available for use as an intravenous contrast agent for MRI. Gadolinium is strongly paramagnetic and causes marked shortening of T1. Areas with breakdown of the blood-brain barrier therefore appear bright on T1-weighted images after gadolinium administration. Serious reactions to gadolinium-based contrast agents are exceedingly rare.

Safety Considerations with MRI

Limitations of MRI include time constraints and safety concerns related to the strong magnetic field. Care must be taken to assess each patient (and attendant) entering the vicinity of the MRI system for metal within or on the body. Many objects, including most surgical clips and orthopedic hardware, do not pose a significant risk to the patient. Cardiac pacemakers and defibrillators, among other devices, are contraindications to MRI. Fatal accidents have occurred. Some aneurysm clips are not MRI-safe. Lists are available regarding metallic implants that are considered safe. Objects to be taken into the vicinity of the magnet are also carefully screened because ferromagnetic objects can become projectiles. Patient cooperation (or at least immobility) is more critical with MRI than CT. Patient monitoring is also more challenging, although not impossible, with MRI.

OTHER IMAGING TECHNIQUES

Sonography (Ultrasound)

Sonography utilizes high-frequency sound generated from a transducer to produce images based on the echoes from internal structures. Homogeneous liquids, such as CSF, create no echoes, whereas changes at tissue boundaries create changes in the resultant echo. Acute hemorrhage is echogenic and is clearly visualized on ultrasound examination. A neoplasm or other mass that is sufficiently different from adjacent brain or spine tissue can also be identified with ultrasound.

Sonography is relatively inexpensive, widely available, and safe. However, a free path must exist for the ultrasound beam. Bone stops the beam completely. For this reason, CNS ultrasound examination is limited primarily to the newborn or young infant. Before the cranial sutures close, the brain can be imaged through the open fontanelles. This is especially useful in premature infants, who are at high risk for intracranial hemorrhage and who must stay in a monitored, protective environment. Ultrasound equipment is easily transported and used at the bedside in the intensive care nursery. Early in life, the spine can also be examined to a limited extent between the immature bones. Portability implies that sonography can also be used for intraoperative localization.

Doppler Ultrasound

Ultrasound is also the basis of vascular imaging using the Doppler technique. This permits a combination of (1) vessel imaging and (2) waveform display. The latter is associated with velocity of blood flow. Doppler ultrasound is commonly used for noninvasive evaluation of the carotid bifurcation. Transcranial Doppler (TCD) is used for evaluation of intracranial arteries. Although spatial resolution is limited at this time, TCD provides valuable blood flow velocity and waveform characteristics (pulsatility) information.

Nuclear Medicine

Several nuclear medicine tests were used for brain imaging before the advent of CT and MRI. Although the use of radionuclide injection and imaging of emitted gamma rays with a gamma camera is now fairly limited for CNS applications, newer techniques are rekindling interest in CNS nuclear medicine applications. At its simplest, nuclear medicine for CNS imaging involves injection of one of several radionuclides, generally compounds containing technetium-99m, while imaging over the neck and head to evaluate for blood flow and distribution. This test still has utility as a supplemental examination in questions of brain death (see Fig. 5–10). Compounds are now available that have some specificity for brain tissue and therefore provide information about perfusion and metabolism. Although the spatial resolution of radionuclide imaging is poor compared with that of CT and MRI, the information is based on physiologic function. The use of special gamma cameras and software enables reconstruction of tomographic slices in SPECT (single-photon emission computed tomography). The special technology significantly improves spatial resolution.

Other Techniques

Various specialized tests are primarily used for research at this time but may be used for clinical purposes where they are available. PET (positron emission tomography) scanning produces images of the brain after compounds are injected that emit positrons. Several agents that are metabolized in the brain and yield information about cerebral metabolic activity can be employed. PET requires the close proximity of a cyclotron to produce the agents, thus limiting availability.

MRI systems can be used for additional tests. The nuclear magnetic resonance spectra from tissue can be acquired (MR spectroscopy), and some information can be gained about relative quantities of compounds such as N-acetylaspartate (NAA, es-sentially found only in neurons), creatine, choline, and lactate. Other specialized MRI techniques include diffusion-weighted imaging.

Functional MR imaging is technically challenging and of intense interest to many researchers. Functional MRI relies on measuring signal intensity differences associated with brain activity, which are thought to be the result of changes in blood oxygenation.

Another approach to functional imaging correlates MR images with magnetoencephalography (MEG). The resulting montage of information is termed *magnetic source imaging* or MSI. The MEG component can evaluate background activity for the equivalent of spikes and slow waves on electroencephalogram (EEG), or it can detect evoked magnetic activity from repeated brain stimulation. Sensory, motor, auditory, and visual centers of the brain can be localized in this manner. Functional imaging of the brain has applications in presurgical mapping and planning, as well as in research.

2

Cranial Trauma

Neuroimaging plays a key role in the management of head trauma. With the current widespread availability of CT, major complications of head trauma can be quickly recognized and treatment altered accordingly. CT, and more recently MRI, have made possible visualization of the effects of cranial trauma that were once inferred or demonstrated only with invasive techniques.

Head injuries may be classified according to whether the skull is penetrated (penetrating injury) or not (closed head injury). Complete imaging assessment of cranial trauma includes not only detection of hemorrhage, but evaluation of mass effect, shift of intracranial structures, and presence of secondary effects such as infarction and hydrocephalus.

EXTRA-AXIAL AND INTRAVENTRICULAR BLOOD

One of the most important reasons for imaging the brain of a patient with a head injury is to recognize extra-axial (subdural and epidural) hematomas. Subdural and epidural hematomas may be life-threatening and are quite accessible for surgical evacuation. Small hematomas may resolve, but follow-up scans are indicated because of the risk of expansion. CT is usually the test of choice for the detection of acute intracranial hemorrhage. Acute hemorrhage is usually dense (bright) on CT. Intermediate window settings on CT can be very helpful to detect blood adjacent to bone (Fig. 2–1). (Note that in addition to the illustrations included in this chapter, several examples of epidural and subdural hematomas of various sizes may be found in Appendix 1.)

Epidural Hematomas

Epidural hematomas usually result from arterial bleeding, often from laceration of the middle meningeal artery by a squamosal temporal bone fracture. Venous or mixed sources, however, may cause epidural hematomas. They may occur without recognized fracture in a minority of cases. Epidural hematomas do not cross sutures. They occur in a variety of locations, including the posterior fossa. Most commonly, however, they occur in the region of the temporal lobe. The classic clinical presentation includes a head injury followed by a lucid interval and subsequent deterioration (Fig. 2–2). This pattern, however, is not reliable for diagnosis and occurs in a minority of patients with epidural hematoma.

On CT, epidural hematomas are localized regions of high attenuation outside the brain (extra-axial), usually with convex margins or a lentiform shape (Figs. 2–2, 2–3). They may cause considerable local mass effect. Prompt evacuation may result in dramatic improvement. An inhomoge-

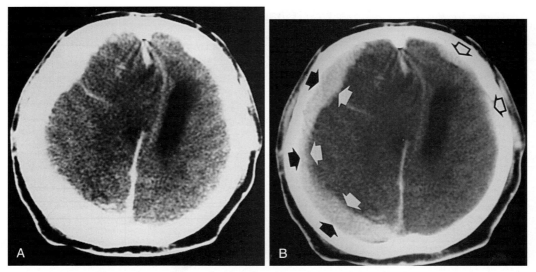

Figure 2–1. Intermediate CT window settings for trauma. *(A)* Routine soft tissue window setting on CT scan of the brain of a trauma patient shows subarachnoid hemorrhage, shift of the midline to the patient's left, and an enlarged (trapped) left lateral ventricle. *(B)* Intermediate window and level settings at the same location enable visualization of blood, which is denser than brain but less dense than skull, in a huge right subdural hematoma *(solid arrows)* and smaller left subdural hematoma *(open arrows)*.

neous appearance has occasionally been described in active hemorrhage. CT, which is easily and quickly obtained, widely available, and sensitive for the detection of acute hemorrhage, is the test of choice. If an MRI scan is obtained for other reasons, epidural hematomas have the same lentiform or biconvex shape as is observed on CT, whereas signal intensity varies depending on the age of the clot.

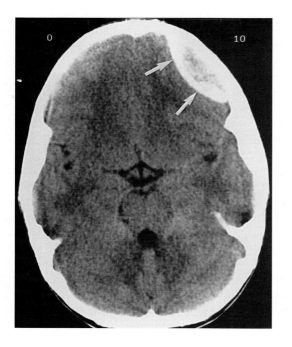

Figure 2–2. Epidural hematoma. CT scan was obtained in a 6-year-old girl who suffered a head injury, had a lucid interval, then became symptomatic. Biconvex, high attenuation, left frontal epidural hematoma is present *(arrows)*.

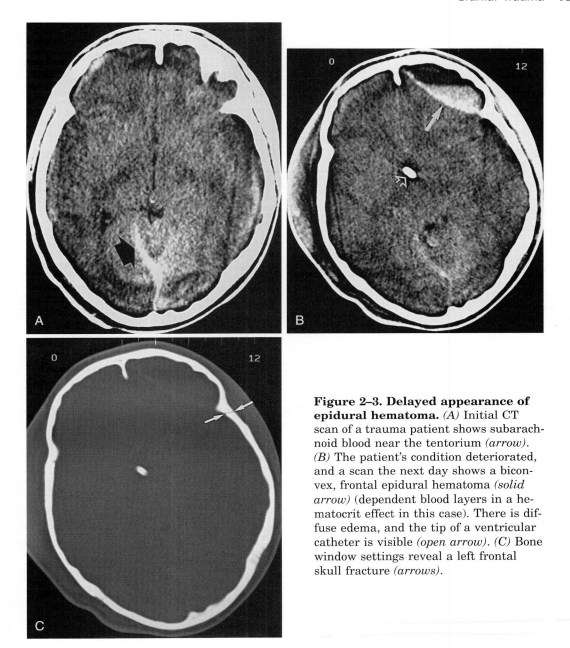

Figure 2–3. Delayed appearance of epidural hematoma. *(A)* Initial CT scan of a trauma patient shows subarachnoid blood near the tentorium *(arrow)*. *(B)* The patient's condition deteriorated, and a scan the next day shows a biconvex, frontal epidural hematoma *(solid arrow)* (dependent blood layers in a hematocrit effect in this case). There is diffuse edema, and the tip of a ventricular catheter is visible *(open arrow)*. *(C)* Bone window settings reveal a left frontal skull fracture *(arrows)*.

Subdural Hematomas

Subdural hematomas are not confined by tight attachment between dura and bone, as are epidural hematomas. They are broader collections of blood, often extending widely across the convexity of a cerebral hemisphere. They may cross suture lines, in contrast to epidural hematomas. In cross-section they appear crescentic on CT or MRI, with the attenuation or signal intensity of blood. Bilateral subdural hematomas may occur (see Fig. 2–1). Mass effect may shift the midline or efface the sulci immediately underlying the hematoma. Subdural hematomas usually result from venous bleeding. Frequently there is underlying parenchymal damage. The most common location is over the cerebral convexities, but interhemispheric and tentorial subdural hematomas

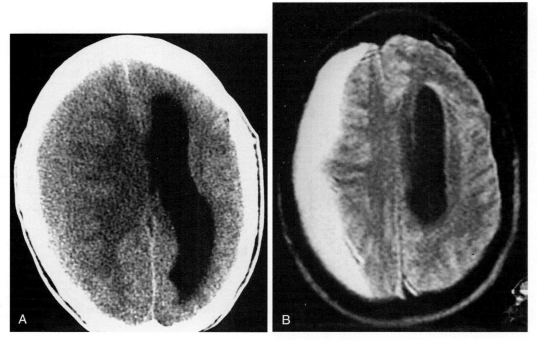

Figure 2–4. Isodense subdural hematoma on CT, and MRI appearance. *(A)* Axial CT shows severe displacement of the gray-white matter junction on the patient's right side. The hematoma is large but isodense with brain. The left lateral ventricle is markedly enlarged because of entrapment at the level of the foramen of Monro from subfalcine herniation. *(B)* Axial long TR/short TE MRI scan performed on the same day shows the hematoma as an obvious area of very bright signal intensity.

also occur. Interhemispheric subdural hematomas in children may be the result of shaking or other abuse.

The imaging appearance of subdural hematomas, like that of other intracranial blood, depends on the age of the hematoma. Acute hemorrhage initially has higher attenuation than brain. Over the following several days to weeks, attenuation of a hematoma decreases until the chronic hematoma is less dense than brain and closer to that of CSF. Between these stages is a period when a hematoma may have very similar attenuation (isodense) to that of brain on CT. The typical evolution of hemorrhage on CT and MRI scans is presented in further detail in Chapter 6. Acute subdural hematomas are usually easily identified with CT (see Figs. 2–1, 2–11). However, subacute subdural hematomas may be more difficult to identify. Attenuation of subacute blood can be very close to that of brain. Mass effect and inward displacement of the cortical gray matter are important clues to

the presence of extra-axial hematomas (Fig. 2–4). The vascular neomembrane that forms around a subdural hematoma demonstrates enhancement if intravenous contrast material is given. Not all subdural hematomas require evacuation. The degree of mass effect and extent of pre-existing cortical atrophy are important factors in assessing the significance of extra-axial hematomas (Fig. 2–5). Imaging studies may be used to document resolution.

Mixed attenuation on CT can result from rebleeding into a chronic subdural hematoma. A mixed pattern is also occasionally observed in acute subdural hematomas, especially large ones.

MRI is more sensitive than CT for the detection of subdural blood, especially small collections and hematomas isodense with brain on CT (see Figs. 2–4, 9–31). As with CT, subdural fluid collections are usually crescentic. Signal intensity depends on a variety of factors, including the evolution of hemoglobin (see Chapter 6).

Subarachnoid and Intraventricular Hemorrhage

Subarachnoid hemorrhage very commonly accompanies head trauma. It is identified as a region of high density on CT within the subarachnoid spaces (the sulci and/or cisterns) (Figs. 2–1, 2–6). Blood in the subarachnoid space alone is not a significant acute problem, although it is among the conditions that can block the arachnoid granulations and lead to convexity-level (communicating) hydrocephalus. MRI is relatively insensitive to subarachnoid hemorrhage.

Intraventricular hemorrhage is also common in head injury. Its primary importance lies in the possibility of subsequent hydrocephalus. A resultant hydrocephalus may be due to obstruction at the level of the cerebral aqueduct or elsewhere within the ventricular system, or because of communicating hydrocephalus from obstruction of arachnoid granulations. Intraventricular hemorrhage often accompanies other types of intracranial hemorrhage (see Fig. 6–2).

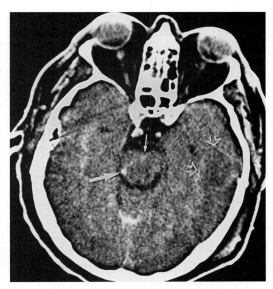

Figure 2–6. Midbrain hemorrhage, contusions, and subarachnoid hemorrhage. CT scan of a man who was in a motor vehicle accident. There is hemorrhage at the dorsolateral midbrain *(large arrow)*, most likely resulting from impact against the tentorium. Low density in the left temporal lobe *(open arrows)* is related to contusions. (Fracture of the left temporal bone was visible on lower slices.) High attenuation of subarachnoid blood is present in the superior cerebellar cistern, sylvian fissure, and interpeduncular fossa *(small arrow).*

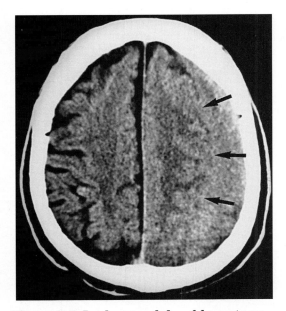

Figure 2–5. Isodense subdural hematoma with minimal mass effect. Axial, nonenhanced CT scan of an elderly man shows loss of sulci on the left side because of an isodense subdural hematoma *(arrows).* Because of the degree of atrophy, there is no midline shift despite the size of the hematoma.

Prominent intracranial hemorrhage that is observed by imaging studies after only minor trauma may be indicative of ruptured aneurysm or arteriovenous malformations (AVM) that caused loss of consciousness and a fall or accident.

INJURY OF THE BRAIN

Penetrating Injury

Injury of the brain can result from penetrating injury or closed head injury. Penetrating injury causes direct trauma to the brain with hemorrhage and edema that may expand. Additional damage may arise from the force of impact. This shock wave injury is most dramatic with gunshot wounds. A risk of infection is always present. CT scan-

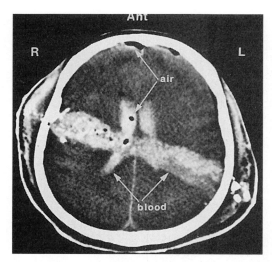

Figure 2–7. Penetrating injury of the head. Nonenhanced CT scan of the head of a gunshot victim. The bullet path is readily visualized because of the high-density blood along the tract. High-density bullet and bone fragments and low density air are visible. (From Mettler F: Essentials of Radiology. Philadelphia, WB Saunders, 1995, p 24.)

The brain opposite the site of the direct blow can receive a contrecoup injury as it in turn strikes the unyielding skull. Contusions are visible as areas of high attenuation on CT (Figs. 2–6, 2–8, 2–9). They may increase in size and number in the initial day or two after injury. Early contusions are detected with greater sensitivity by MRI. Deep cerebral gray matter hemorrhage can occur with closed head trauma.

Shearing Injury

A second important type of closed head injury is severe diffuse axonal injury or shearing injury. This results from rotational or deceleration forces on the brain. The differing physical properties (density) of gray and white matter result in differing rates of deceleration or acceleration and cause shearing. Common locations include the subcortical gray-white junction and the corpus callosum. Small areas of hemorrhage and/or edema result, which can be observed on CT or, with greater sensitivity, on MRI

ning is useful to evaluate hemorrhage, other brain damage (edema or herniation), and presence of foreign bodies (Fig. 2–7). Vascular damage can cause infarction distant from the missile tract (Chapter 5). Contrast studies may be necessary at a later time if abscess is suspected.

Contusion

Closed head injury is a major cause of death and morbidity. Contusion of the brain is initially manifested on CT as a region of low density mixed with small areas of high density. Edema often increases over several days before resolving. The amount of blood visible on CT also frequently increases during the first day. Large parenchymal hematomas can cause considerable local mass effect. Contusions are often superficial in location and are especially common where the brain lies against underlying bone. The anterior temporal lobes and inferior frontal lobes are commonly involved. Coup and contrecoup injuries can often be identified. The coup injury is at the site of skull impact, where bone strikes the underlying brain.

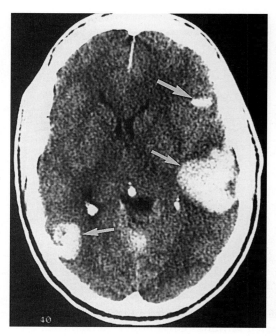

Figure 2–8. Cortical contusions. Large, hemorrhagic cortical contusions are visible on nonenhanced CT as areas of high attenuation *(arrows)*. Larger contusions on the left cause mass effect, with left-to-right shift.

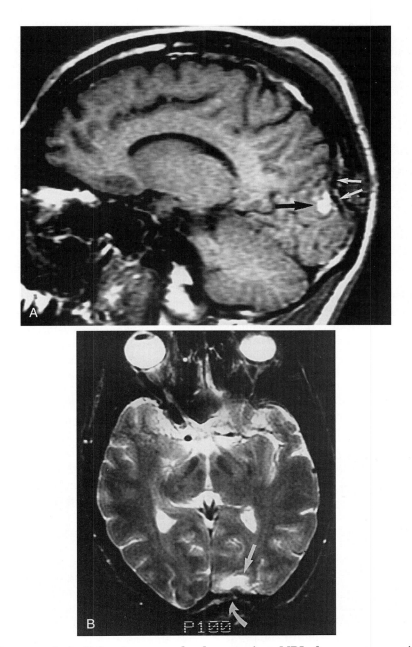

Figure 2–9. Depressed skull fracture, cerebral contusion. MRI of a young man with depressed skull fracture. *(A)* Sagittal, nonenhanced T1WI shows the inwardly displaced area of bone *(white arrows)*. Of greater importance is high signal intensity of subacute hemorrhage *(black arrow)* in the underlying occipital lobe. *(B)* Axial T2WI also shows the fracture *(curved arrow)* and high signal of blood and edema in the occipital lobe *(straight arrow)*. The superior sagittal sinus is also at risk for occlusion because of the location of the fracture, but MRI showed it not to be occluded.

(Fig. 2–10). Multiple lesions are usually present. The neurologic sequelae of this injury are often out of proportion to the neuroimaging abnormalities. Extensive areas of diffuse axonal injury are associated with a poor prognosis for full recovery.

INTRACRANIAL HERNIATIONS

Types of Herniations

Mass effect within the closed space of the cranium can have devastating secondary effects. The initial response to swelling or hemorrhage within the head is compression of adjacent structures. Shifts of the ventricular system and the midline structures are important clues to the presence of mass effect.

Greater shifts of structures across the midline cause herniation under the falx cerebri (subfalcine herniation). Dilatation of the contralateral ventricle can accompany compression of the ipsilateral ventricle, as the foramen of Monro is obstructed. The anterior cerebral artery can be compressed under the stiff falx, leading to ischemia or infarction. Increasing supratentorial pres-

sure and edema lead to downward swelling. The uncus can be pushed against the brainstem, shifting the brainstem, and cranial nerves and arteries can be compressed. Uncal herniation typically causes third cranial nerve compression and ipsilateral pupillary dilatation. Herniation through the tentorium can also cause posterior cerebral artery compression and occipital lobe ischemia or infarction. The cisterns around the midbrain become effaced. Eventually, transtentorial herniation causes severe compromise of the brainstem. Compression and shearing of perforating arteries from the basilar artery can lead to secondary brainstem (Duret) hemorrhage. Much less commonly, mass effect within the posterior fossa can cause upward herniation through the tentorial notch.

Downward herniation of the cerebellar tonsils also occurs with increasing shifts of the posterior fossa contents. When the intracranial pressure exceeds that of the arterial system, perfusion of the brain effectively ceases and brain death results.

Imaging of Herniation

Both CT and MRI can reveal the changes described earlier. Attention should be directed to alterations in the ventricular contour, midline shift, effacement of cortical sulci, and effacement of the cisterns around the base of the brain (Fig. 2–11). Duret hemorrhages are typically identified in the central midbrain (Fig. 2–12).

Imaging studies can play an important complementary role to the clinical examination in decision-making about medical or surgical intervention for intracranial mass effect. Similar changes accompany other types of intracranial masses, such as tumors or abscesses, but rapid changes are tolerated much more poorly than slow processes. Low-grade neoplasms, for example, can cause considerable distortion of adjacent structures before causing symptoms.

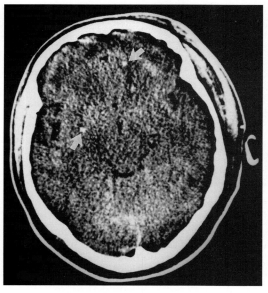

Figure 2–10. Shearing injury. CT scan of a young man who was in a motor vehicle accident. Several small bright foci *(arrows)* represent hemorrhagic shearing injury (diffuse axonal injury) within the brain.

SKULL FRACTURES

Skull fractures are common following major trauma. However, with the exception of penetrating trauma and depressed skull frac-

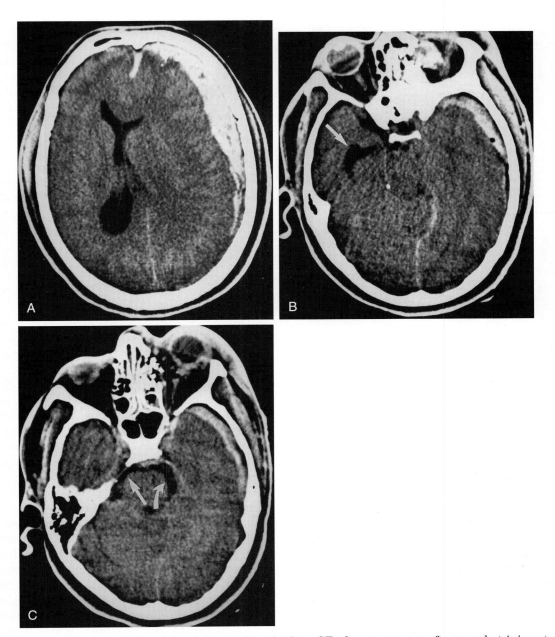

Figure 2–11. Large subdural hematoma, herniation. CT of a young man after gunshot injury to the head. *(A)* Axial CT at the level of the body of the lateral ventricles shows a large, left subdural hematoma. The left frontal cortex is displaced medially. The midline is shifted to the right (subfalcine herniation). Small foci of higher density are bullet fragments. *(B)* At the level of the temporal horn, the subdural hematoma is again visible, with a small bubble of air. The right temporal horn *(arrow)* is dilated because the right lateral ventricle is obstructed at the foramen of Monro due to subfalcine herniation. The left uncus (most medial temporal lobe) is herniated to the right, and the entire brainstem is shifted to the right. *(C)* At the level of the top of the fourth ventricle, shift of the brainstem to the right is again visible, with a larger cistern present to the left of the pons *(curved arrow)* than to the right *(straight arrow)*.

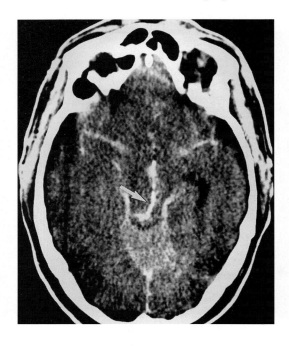

Figure 2–12. Duret hemorrhage. Axial, nonenhanced CT scan of the brain of a man shortly after surgical evacuation of a large subdural hematoma that caused transtentorial herniation. Midbrain Duret hemorrhage is present *(arrow)*, as is subarachnoid hemorrhage.

tures (Fig. 2–13), the presence or absence of a fracture does not alter management. Regardless of the presence of fracture, it is the condition of the underlying brain that is important.

Numerous reports have confirmed that skull films are *not* routinely necessary or indicated for evaluation of head injury. If clinical indications exist for imaging of a patient who has suffered head injury, CT is the most appropriate first test. Absence of fracture on skull films does not exclude major intracranial injury, and the presence of a nondisplaced fracture does not necessarily imply significant injury to the brain. CT, however, reveals acute intracranial hematomas that require urgent intervention. MRI is more sensitive than CT for small extra-axial hematomas, cortical contusions, and axonal or shearing injuries and may be helpful in some cases (see Fig. 2–9). Bone windows on CT, on which the image is presented in a manner to highlight bone rather than soft tissue detail, often show fractures (see Fig. 2–3C). Fractures that lie primarily parallel to the plane of scanning may be missed on CT (Fig. 2–14). Although a nondisplaced linear skull fracture does not need specific care, a fracture crossing the middle meningeal artery may provide a clue to in-

creased risk of epidural hematoma (see Fig. 2–3). On occasion, the scout or localizing image obtained with CT may reveal a fracture that is not visible on the axial images themselves (see Fig. 2–14).

CSF Leaks

Fractures into the skull base, paranasal sinuses, or petrous temporal bones are associated with increased risk of CSF leak and infection. Such fractures may be very difficult to identify on CT, sometimes requiring high-resolution, thin-section technique. The presence of blood or air-fluid levels within the sphenoid or frontal sinuses or mastoid air cells signals the possibility of occult fracture.

Several imaging techniques are available to demonstrate CSF leaks. When the existence of such a leak requires confirmation, injection of a radionuclide into the subarachnoid space can be performed, with subsequent measurement of activity from pledgets placed in the nose. More direct demonstration of the site of a leak can be obtained with T2-weighted MR images in the coronal plane, which show high-signal-intensity fluid extending contiguously from the intracranial space to the extracranial

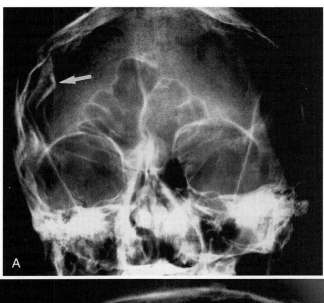

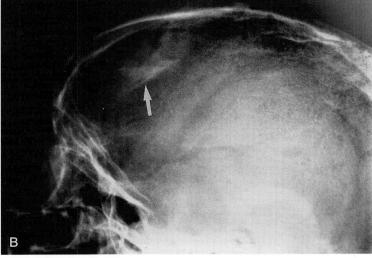

Figure 2–13. Depressed skull fracture. *(A)* Depressed right frontal skull fracture *(arrow)* is easily visible on the AP view. *(B)* On lateral view, the fracture is manifested primarily by increased density *(arrow)*. Skull radiographs are *not* indicated for detection of fractures. CT provides this information, as well as information regarding the brain parenchyma.

space against a background of low-signal-intensity bone. Coronal thin-section CT performed after intrathecal injection of iodinated contrast can also demonstrate a CSF leak, but it is a more invasive technique.

Temporal Bone Fractures

Fractures of the petrous portion of the temporal bone are often classified according to their relationship to the long axis of the bone—i.e., either longitudinal or transverse.

The former is more common. Facial nerve damage occurs more often with transverse fractures. Inner ear damage and ossicular disruption are other consequences of temporal bone injury. Thin-section CT is the best imaging test for temporal bone trauma (Fig. 2–15).

Growing Fractures

A growing fracture is a late complication of skull fracture in children. Laceration of the

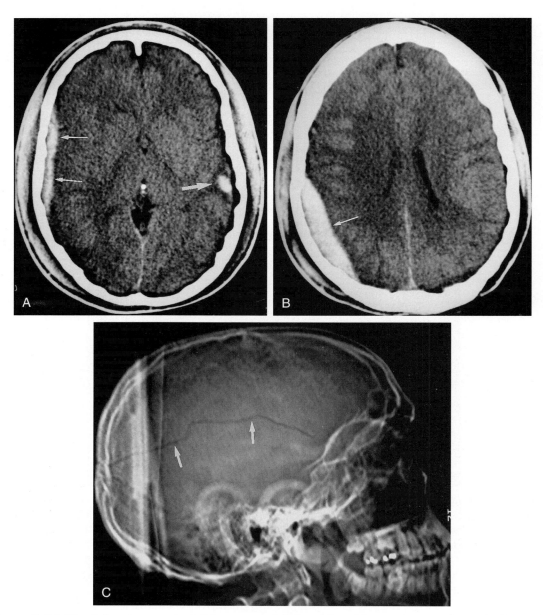

Figure 2–14. Skull fracture not visible on axial CT; epidural hematoma and cortical contusion. *(A)* CT scan of the head after trauma. There is a right-sided extra-axial hematoma *(small arrows)* with a contrecoup cortical contusion *(large arrow)*. *(B)* The epidural hematoma is large and has a more typical biconvex configuration *(arrow)* on a higher section. A fracture could not be detected on the axial images with bone windows, but the digital scout image for the CT *(C)* clearly shows a long fracture *(arrows)*, which overlies the epidural hematoma. The fracture lies nearly in the same plane as the CT slices.

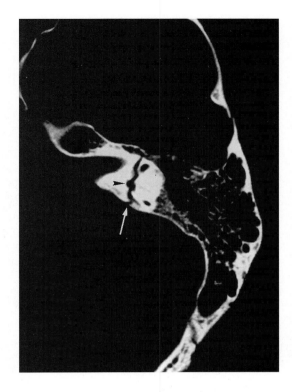

Figure 2–15. Transverse fracture of the petrous portion of the temporal bone. High-resolution axial CT scan of a young man who was in an automobile accident. A fracture *(arrow)* extends in AP direction across the petrous portion of the left temporal bone, crossing the common crus of the semicircular canals *(arrowhead)*. Soft tissue density, probably blood, is present within the epitympanum and some mastoid air cells. Temporal bone fractures are named according to the long axis of the temporal bone; in this case, the fracture is transverse to the long axis.

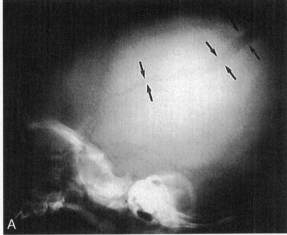

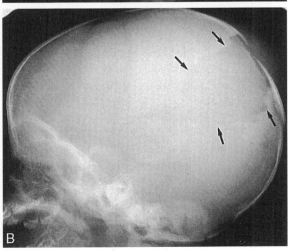

Figure 2–16. Growing skull fracture (leptomeningeal cyst). *(A)* Initial lateral skull radiograph shows a linear, parietal skull fracture *(arrows)*. *(B)* On a film taken several weeks later, the skull defect is much larger *(arrows)*. (From Mettler F: Essentials of Radiology. Philadelphia, WB Saunders, 1995, p 382.)

dura mater results in growth of a leptomeningeal cyst, causing an expanding defect in
the skull (Fig. 2–16).

LATE EFFECTS OF CRANIAL TRAUMA

Late sequelae of cerebral trauma include
atrophy, focal volume loss, and gliosis. MRI
is more sensitive than CT for showing old
areas of hemorrhage and gliosis. Hydrocephalus can also develop, as discussed earlier, which is readily observed with either
CT or MRI.

CONCLUSION

Imaging of head trauma is important in an
acute care setting, especially when surgery
is contemplated, and complications of
trauma are suspected. CT is very sensitive
for acute hemorrhage and shows bone well.
MRI is sensitive for all stages of hemorrhage (except subarachnoid hemorrhage),
for shearing injury, and for edema and contusion. The two modalities are thus complementary for evaluation of cranial injury. A
combination of studies, used at appropriate
times, yields the most information.

3

Infections of the Brain and Meninges

Infections of the central nervous system are very serious. Untreated, they can have grave consequences. Detection of infections is imperative because treatment is often possible. Promptly diagnosing infection and identifying the agent so that proper therapy can be administered are the highest priorities. Imaging may detect processes such as abscess and encephalitis, may localize focal conditions, and may help demonstrate the progress or resolution of infections.

MENINGITIS

Bacterial meningitis is common and is associated with serious morbidity. A variety of bacteria can be responsible; the most common types are dependent on the patient's age. For example, in the newborn, group B streptococcus and *Escherichia coli* predominate. *Haemophilus influenzae* is the most common cause in infants and children. Meningococcal meningitis is especially frequent in teenagers and young adults, whereas pneumococcal meningitis is most common in adults. Although empiric therapy may occasionally be necessary, identification of an organism is desirable to ensure appropriate treatment in each case.

The key diagnostic evidence in suspected meningitis comes from cerebrospinal fluid analysis and culture; imaging has an adjunctive role only. If there is a question of increased intracranial pressure that could make lumbar puncture dangerous, CT is often obtained initially. Inflammatory exudates may obscure the subarachnoid cisterns on noncontrasted CT, whereas meningeal enhancement may be observed on CT or MRI following intravenous contrast material administration (Fig. 3–1). Lack of visible contrast enhancement does not exclude meningitis. Other conditions, including prior surgery, can also cause meningeal enhancement.

Complications of Meningitis

Imaging is important for evaluating complications of meningitis. Communicating hydrocephalus may occur, and ventricular size is readily followed with CT or MRI (Fig. 3–2). Inflammation can lead to vasculitis or vasospasm, with subsequent ischemia or infarction. CT or MRI is useful in revealing ischemic changes, although MRI has greater sensitivity. Angiography is usually reserved for unusual cases in which vasculitis must be confirmed, with subsequent alteration of therapy. Subdural fluid collections (hygromas) (Fig. 3–3) are especially common with *H. influenzae* meningitis. These hygromas usually resolve, but large collections infrequently are associated with

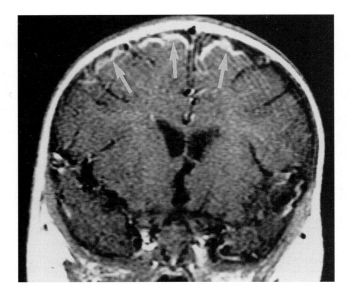

Figure 3–1. Pneumococcal meningitis. MRI (coronal T1WI) in a 6-month-old child demonstrates scattered areas of <u>meningeal enhancement</u> over the frontal and temporal lobes *(arrows)*.

significant mass or pressure effect on the underlying brain. Infection can lead to a subdural empyema, which may require surgical drainage if it serves as a reservoir of continued infection (Fig. 3–4).

Spread of infection can occur. Ventriculitis occurs when the ependyma or lining of the ventricles becomes infected. Enhancement along the margins of the ventricles may be the only imaging evidence. Epidural empyema is uncommon but is also very serious. This localized infection in the epidural space

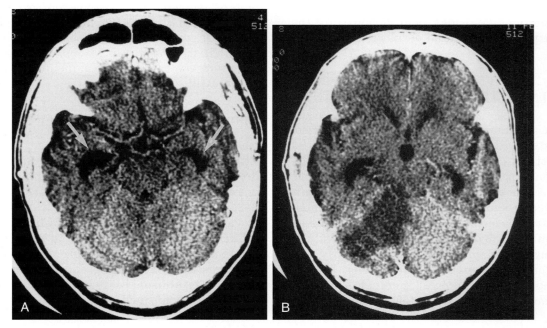

Figure 3–2. Complications of meningitis. *(A)* Initial noncontrasted CT scan in an adult with meningitis shows enlarged temporal horns *(arrows)*, indicating <u>mild hydrocephalus</u>. *(B)* A contrast-enhanced scan taken 1 week later reveals low density associated with right cerebellar hemisphere infarction, in addition to hydrocephalus.

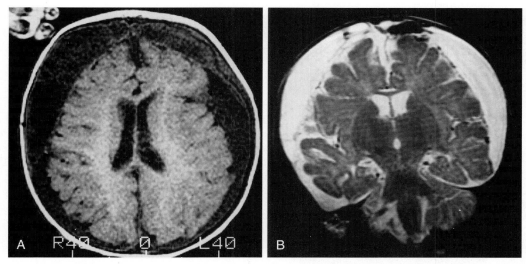

Figure 3–3. Subdural effusions following meningitis. MRI of a child who had a previous episode of meningitis. *(A)* Axial T1WI and *(B)* coronal T2WI show severe volume loss of the brain and prominent extra-axial fluid collections around the brain.

demonstrates contrast enhancement. Cortical vein thrombosis followed by venous infarction may complicate empyema formation.

INFECTION OF THE BRAIN

Cerebritis and Pyogenic Abscess

Infection of the brain itself begins as cerebritis. Cerebritis is initially detected as an area of low attenuation edema on CT or of high signal intensity on intermediate and T2-weighted MRI. The pattern of contrast enhancement varies. With time, bacterial infection progresses to abscess formation (Table 3–1). A collagenous wall forms, which

is usually fairly thin and uniform. Frequently the wall is thinnest on the side nearest the lateral ventricle. Considerable surrounding vasogenic edema is often present (Fig. 3–5). The central fluid attenuation or signal intensity and surrounding edema are readily observed on CT or MRI. The wall may be visualized as an area of high density on CT or lower signal intensity on MRI. A well-defined ring-like pattern of enhancement appears after contrast material administration. Abscess is *not* the only cause of a ring-enhancing pattern in the brain; primary or metastatic neoplasm, infarction, and resolving hematomas also commonly have such a pattern of enhancement. Conditions such as thrombosed aneu-

TABLE 3–1. **Stages of Abscess Formation**

Stage	Characteristics/Time Course
Early cerebritis	About 3–5 days; infection not localized or encapsulated
Late cerebritis	Up to 10–14 days; areas of necrosis coalesce into a central zone; a ring of inflammatory cells forms but is not yet a capsule
Early abscess	Beginning about 2 weeks; a thin, collagenous capsule forms
Late abscess	May last for many weeks; a complete capsule is present, with three layers: inner layer of granulation tissue and macrophages, middle collagenous layer, and outer gliotic layer

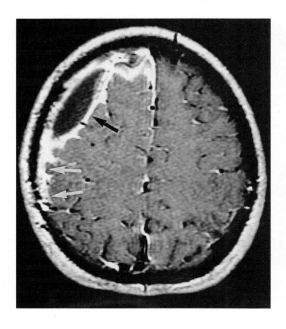

Figure 3–4. Extra-axial empyema. Subdural empyema was present in this young man with meningitis. Note the right frontal, elliptical fluid collection with enhancing rim on post-gadolinium T1WI *(black arrow)*. Nearby meningeal enhancement is also present *(white arrows)*.

rysm or arteriovenous malformation (AVM) and (on MRI) multiple sclerosis plaque may also have this pattern (see Table 4–1).

Pyogenic abscesses are most often the result of hematogenous spread of infection. Contiguous or direct spread of infection from sinusitis, otitis, or mastoiditis can also lead to a brain abscess. It is important to inspect these potential extracranial sources of infection via CT or MRI (see Fig. 3–5). In addition to pyogenic sources, ring-enhancing patterns with infection may also occur with tuberculosis (TB), fungal infections, protozoal infections (*Toxoplasma*), and parasitic infection. Abscesses from nonpyogenic infections are often more irregular in appearance than the thin, uniform capsule of pyogenic abscesses.

Encephalitis

Viral infection of the brain results in encephalitis. One of the most common types is herpes encephalitis, which in adults most frequently results from herpes simplex type 1. This necrotizing, hemorrhagic encephalitis represents a medical emergency. The temporal and frontal lobes are most commonly involved. Bilateral but asymmetric involvement is very common. Contrast enhancement usually develops but may be patchy or gyriform. Hemorrhage occurs in

herpes encephalitis but is often not present initially. Edema, contrast enhancement, and hemorrhage may be present on CT, but MRI is the test of choice, especially in the early stages of encephalitis. Because of the high morbidity of encephalitis and availability of a specific antiviral therapy, the possibility of herpes infection should always be kept in mind. Abnormal signal intensity on MRI in the temporal or frontal lobe, especially with bilateral involvement, enhancement, or evidence of hemorrhage, suggests herpes encephalitis (Fig. 3–6).

Other Infectious Agents: TB, Fungi, Parasites, and Others

The incidence of CNS TB is increasing because of higher numbers of immunocompromised patients and overall spread of the disease. It is often but not always associated with pulmonary TB. TB meningitis is typically a basilar meningitis. Communicating hydrocephalus and vasculitis are common sequelae. Contrast-enhanced CT or MRI demonstrates enhancement in the basilar cisterns (Fig. 3–7). Vasculitis results in areas of ischemia or infarction, as the vessels traversing the exudate in the basilar cisterns are in turn affected. Enhancement of the ependyma indicates ependymitis. Focal infection may also be present, with one or

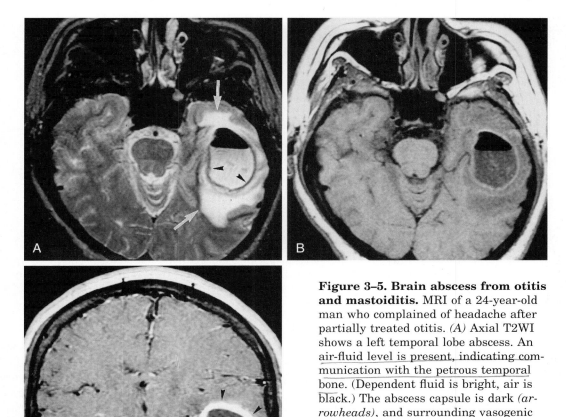

Figure 3–5. Brain abscess from otitis and mastoiditis. MRI of a 24-year-old man who complained of headache after partially treated otitis. *(A)* Axial T2WI shows a left temporal lobe abscess. An air-fluid level is present, indicating communication with the petrous temporal bone. (Dependent fluid is bright, air is black.) The abscess capsule is dark *(arrowheads)*, and surrounding vasogenic edema is bright *(white arrows)*. *(B)* On precontrast axial T1WI, both fluid within the abscess and edema fluid are dark gray. The capsule is slightly hyperintense, a common appearance for an abscess capsule on T1WI. *(C)* Coronal postgadolinium T1WI shows intense contrast enhancement of the capsule *(arrowheads)*, communication between the brain and temporal bone, and enhancement within the middle ear space and mastoid air cells *(white arrow)*.

more tuberculomas (Fig. 3–8). On imaging, tuberculomas have the appearance of a ring-enhancing mass. Central calcification or enhancement and a peripheral ring can cause a target appearance. Active infection is associated with surrounding edema. Old TB lesions are often calcified and have no associated edema.

Fungal infections are uncommon in the immunocompetent patient. Pulmonary disease, with subsequent hematogenous spread, is the most common source. Coccidioidomycosis, histoplasmosis, and blastomycosis occur in specific geographic regions of the United States and often result in pulmo-

nary disease. CNS involvement, which is much less common, usually results in chronic meningoencephalitis (Fig. 3–9). Coccidioidomycosis often results in hydrocephalus; cerebritis, infarction, and granulomas may also occur. Other fungal diseases are discussed later in the section on the immunocompromised patient.

Infection of humans with ova of the pork parasite, *Taenia solium,* results in cysticercosis. This is the most common parasitic CNS infection in the United States and is endemic in many other areas of the world. Encysted larvae within muscle have a characteristic calcified appearance (rice grains).

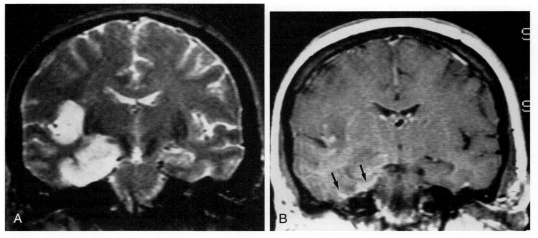

Figure 3–6. Herpes encephalitis. *(A)* Coronal T2WI shows markedly increased signal intensity along the medial and inferior right temporal lobe and along the insular cortex. *(B)* On a coronal contrasted T1WI, there is faint contrast enhancement along the inferomedial temporal cortex *(arrows).*

Infection of the CNS results in a complex series of changes, and various locations can be involved. Table 3–2 summarizes the stages through which parenchymal cysts pass. These cysts initially cause little inflammation, but the dying organism incites an inflammatory reaction (Fig. 3–10). With time the cysts shrink, ultimately leaving only small calcifications (Fig. 3–11). Although a single lesion passes through these stages, lesions in various stages can be simultaneously observed within the brain. Antiparasitic therapy is available but carries some risk of accelerating the inflammatory damage that arises from dying cysticerci. Cysts can also occur within the ventricles. These can be difficult to detect; they are best visualized on MRI. Intraventricular cysts can lead to CSF obstruction and hydrocephalus. Cysts within the suba-

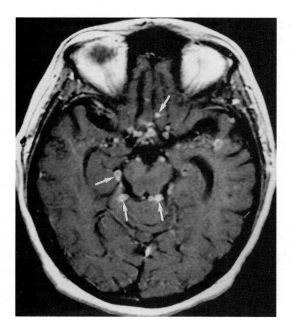

Figure 3–7. Tuberculous meningitis in AIDS. MRI scan (axial post-gadolinium T1WI) from a 35-year-old with headaches shows multiple, small, ring-enhancing abscesses in the subarachnoid spaces around the base of the brain *(arrows).*

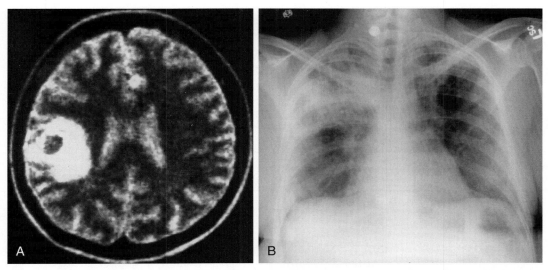

Figure 3–8. Tuberculoma in a patient with pulmonary TB. *(A)* Axial intermediate-weighted MRI shows a right cerebral mass with surrounding high signal intensity of vasogenic edema. *(B)* Extensive chest opacities were present on chest radiograph, with right upper lobe predominance.

rachnoid spaces are also best detected with MRI. A racemose form (resembling a cluster of grapes and without a scolex) is particularly common in this location (see Fig. 3–10*B*).

Neurosyphilis causes both vascular disease (with areas of infarction visible on CT or MRI), and gummas, which appear as mass lesions.

Acute disseminated encephalomyelitis (ADEM) is a rare complication of viral infection or vaccination. The disease is thought to be the result of an autoimmune process. Perivenular demyelination results in white

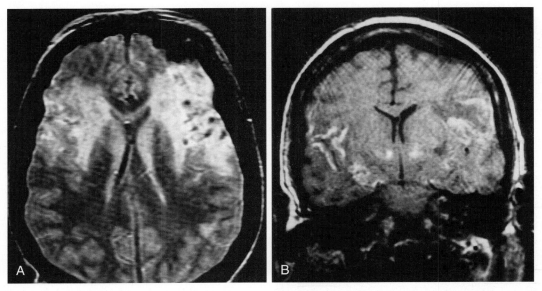

Figure 3–9. Coccidioidomycosis meningitis. *(A)* On MRI, an axial intermediate-weighted image (long TR, short TE) demonstrates extensive cortical edema around the sylvian fissures bilaterally. *(B)* On a post-gadolinium coronal T1WI, there is enhancement in a gyral pattern and in a few deeper locations.

TABLE 3–2. **Stages of Neurocysticercosis (Escobar Classification)**

Stage	Characteristics of Parenchymal Cysticerci
Vesicular	Cyst is visible, occasionally with a scolex visible as an eccentric nodule within the cyst; there is little surrounding inflammation
Colloidal vesicular	Dying organism incites inflammation
	Ring-enhancement pattern present
	Surrounding edema within the brain
Granular nodular	Cyst shrinks further, begins to calcify
Nodular calcified	Cyst is no longer visible
	Only a small calcification remains

A parenchymal lesion takes an average of 5 years (range 2–10 years) to pass through all four stages. Inflammatory response of the brain occurs when the parasite dies.

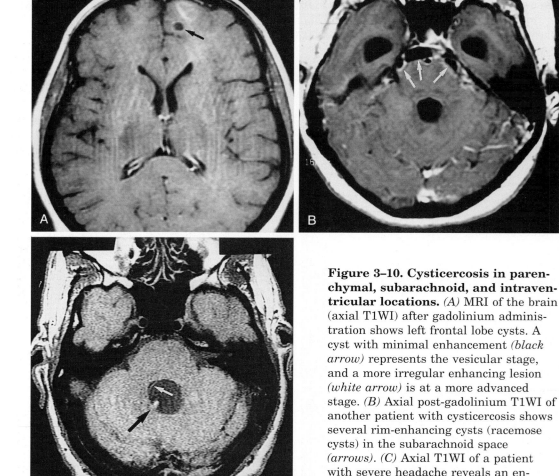

Figure 3–10. Cysticercosis in parenchymal, subarachnoid, and intraventricular locations. *(A)* MRI of the brain (axial T1WI) after gadolinium administration shows left frontal lobe cysts. A cyst with minimal enhancement *(black arrow)* represents the vesicular stage, and a more irregular enhancing lesion *(white arrow)* is at a more advanced stage. *(B)* Axial post-gadolinium T1WI of another patient with cysticercosis shows several rim-enhancing cysts (racemose cysts) in the subarachnoid space *(arrows)*. *(C)* Axial T1WI of a patient with severe headache reveals an enlarged fourth ventricle. An intraventricular cyst fills most of the fourth ventricle, causing hydrocephalus. Part of the wall of the cyst is visible *(white arrow)*. The nodule along the wall of the cyst *(black arrow)* is the scolex, or head, of the parasite.

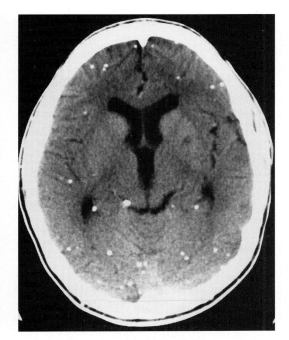

Figure 3–11. Cysticercosis. Nonenhanced CT of a young man with seizures shows innumerable calcifications. Many lie within sulci or on the surface of the brain and represent calcified subarachnoid cysts. Mild communicating hydrocephalus is present.

mon with HIV infection. However, diseases previously considered rare are frequently diagnosed in this group.

HIV Infection

Whereas secondary infections are the usual problem elsewhere in the body, the CNS is often the subject of direct infection by HIV, with resultant clinical dementia. The most common imaging finding of primary HIV infection is atrophy. White matter lesions are also common (Fig. 3–12). Enhancement of these lesions is uncommon.

Progressive Multifocal Leukoencephalopathy

Progressive multifocal leukoencephalopathy (PML) is the result of infection with, or reactivation of, a papovavirus (JC virus). As the name indicates, the course is progressive. Imaging abnormalities are more readily detected on MRI than on CT (Fig. 3–13). Increased T2-weighted signal intensity on MRI or low attenuation on CT is seen in the white matter. PML often appears first in

matter abnormalities that can resemble those of multiple sclerosis on MRI. Subcortical white matter lesions are typically present, but deep white matter and infratentorial lesions may also occur. Lyme disease of the CNS can have a similar appearance.

THE IMMUNOCOMPROMISED PATIENT

Diagnosis and treatment of the immunocompromised patient present some of the greatest challenges facing medicine today. Growing numbers of organ transplant recipients, who are surviving longer, and the increasing population with human immunodeficiency virus (HIV) infection often present with CNS infections. A different set of diseases emerges, when compared with those observed in the immunocompetent patient. Pyogenic infection with abscess is uncom-

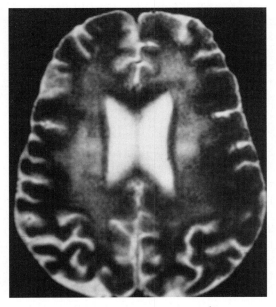

Figure 3–12. HIV infection of the brain. MRI (axial T2WI) of a 38-year-old man with AIDS shows atrophy (prominent ventricles and sulci) and patchy, extensive regions of increased signal intensity in the cerebral white matter.

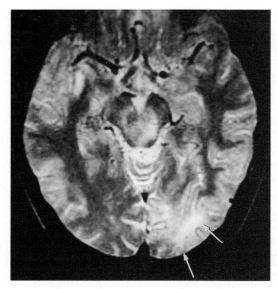

Figure 3–13. <u>Progressive multifocal leu-koencephalopathy (PML)</u>. MRI of a 30-year-old man with AIDS and progressive neurologic deterioration. <u>Axial T2WI shows high signal intensity in the left occipital, subcortical white matter</u> *(arrows)*. The midbrain is also involved. There was <u>no enhancement after gadolinium administration.</u> Autopsy confirmed PML.

the subcortical white matter, but deep white matter involvement is also frequently observed on imaging studies. A posterior parietal or occipital location was considered most common in the past, but greater variation in location and appearance is observed with HIV infection. Enhancement is rare.

Toxoplasmosis

Specific therapy is not currently available for PML or HIV viral infection. Imaging studies are generally obtained for the purpose of detecting treatable conditions. The most common of these is toxoplasmosis. Typical locations are <u>subcortical and within the basal ganglia,</u> but the infection can occur elsewhere in the brain parenchyma. A typical abscess appearance or more solid enhancement may be observed. Follow-up scans can be critical in evaluating the response to treatment (Fig. 3–14). <u>If empiric therapy is ineffective, other diagnoses such as primary CNS lymphoma become much more likely.</u>

Primary CNS lymphoma, discussed further in Chapter 4, can be very difficult to distinguish from toxoplasmosis at times. Ring-like or solid enhancement can be seen, and the two often occur in similar locations. A periventricular location is common but is only part of a more widespread distribution. Failure to respond to therapy for toxoplasmosis is often the most helpful imaging and clinical evidence in favor of lymphoma. The possibility of CNS lymphoma, as well as infection, must be considered when enhancing masses are detected in an immunocompromised patient.

Cytomegalovirus

Cytomegalovirus (CMV) infection of the brain seldom occurs in adults with an intact immune system but is not uncommon in immunocompromised patients. Atrophy is often observed. White matter changes may be similar in appearance to those of primary HIV infection or PML. Periventricular involvement is common with CMV encephalitis, and calcification is seen in congenital infections but not in adult-onset disease.

Fungal and Granulomatous Infection

Fungal infections and tuberculosis (see Fig. 3–7) are also common in immunocompromised patients. They are much less frequent, but not unknown, in immunocompetent patients. Cryptococcosis results in a chronic meningitis. Meningeal enhancement or enhancing parenchymal lesions can occur, and cystic lesions in the basal ganglia are particularly common in cryptococcosis (Fig. 3–15). The "cysts" represent dilated perivascular (Virchow-Robin) CSF spaces and gelatinous pseudocysts. Other fungal infections, such as from *Nocardia* and *Candida,* can cause parenchymal infection and meningitis as well.

Mucormycosis and aspergillosis are rare infections that occur primarily as paranasal sinus disease in diabetic or immunocompromised patients. They can be very invasive, eroding into blood vessels and into the brain itself. Blood-borne aspergillosis can also seed the brain and lead to necrotizing disease.

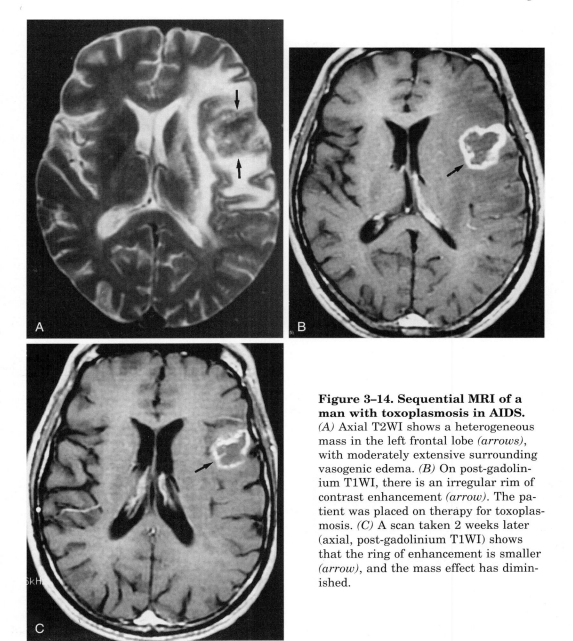

Figure 3–14. Sequential MRI of a man with toxoplasmosis in AIDS. *(A)* Axial T2WI shows a heterogeneous mass in the left frontal lobe *(arrows)*, with moderately extensive surrounding vasogenic edema. *(B)* On post-gadolinium T1WI, there is an irregular rim of contrast enhancement *(arrow)*. The patient was placed on therapy for toxoplasmosis. *(C)* A scan taken 2 weeks later (axial, post-gadolinium T1WI) shows that the ring of enhancement is smaller *(arrow)*, and the mass effect has diminished.

PERINATAL INFECTIONS

A specific set of infectious diseases is frequently associated with prenatal or perinatal infections. Clinical sequelae range from mild impairment to seizures to profound developmental delays. Although these diseases can also occur in adults and older children, the imaging appearance, as well as the clinical manifestations, often differ when infection is acquired in utero or during infancy (Table 3–3).

Cytomegalovirus (CMV) infection is the most common congenital CNS infection. CMV has an affinity for the germinal matrix. The calcifications observed with CMV are often in a periventricular location. Atrophy and neuronal migration abnormalities can also occur (see Chapter 9). Toxoplasmosis acquired in utero (the second most com-

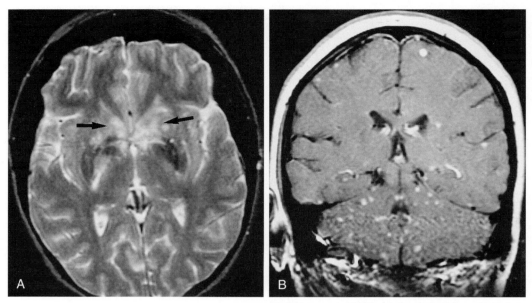

Figure 3–15. Cryptococcal meningitis. *(A)* MRI of a 32-year-old woman with cryptococcosis (axial T2WI) demonstrates several areas of high signal intensity in the basal ganglia *(arrows)*, a common location of cryptococcal pseudocysts in the perivascular spaces. *(B)* Axial post-gadolinium image shows numerous areas of enhancement as well, many of which lie within sulci. These are leptomeningeal and parenchymal microabscesses from hematogenous spread.

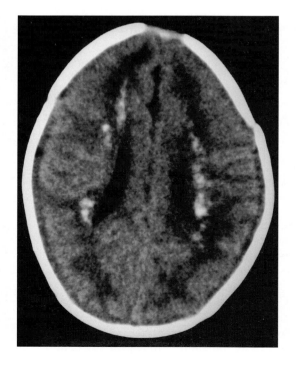

Figure 3–16. Congenital infection. Nonenhanced CT of the brain of a newborn shows extensive calcifications around the lateral ventricles and more peripherally. Basal ganglia calcifications were visible on a lower slice. (This was congenital rubella in a child of an immigrant. Congenital rubella is now rare because of immunization. Toxoplasmosis and CMV are much more common causes of neonatal calcifications in the brain.)

TABLE 3–3. **Congenital CNS Infections**

CMV
Toxoplasmosis
Herpes
HIV
Rubella
Syphilis
(TORCH is a commonly used acronym for
   congenital infections of the brain, including
   *TO*xoplasmosis, *R*ubella, *C*MV, and *H*erpes.)

mon congenital CNS infection) often results in more scattered parenchymal calcifications. Congenital rubella, now rare, can also cause calcifications and atrophy (Fig. 3–16).

Herpes simplex type 1 or type 2 can infect neonates. Type 2 herpes transmitted during delivery is more common. Severe encephalomalacia can result, which is often widespread in extent. The temporal and frontal lobe predominance, characteristic in adults, is absent in neonatal infection.

HIV infection is also somewhat different in infants. Atrophy occurs, but subsequent calcification is common, unlike the condition in adults. However, the calcification is usually not observed in the first year of life.

For the initial evaluation of suspected congenital infection, CT can be helpful because of its increased sensitivity to calcifications. MRI, however, has advantages over CT for the detection of neuronal migration abnormalities.

4

Neoplasms of the Brain

EVALUATION OF MASS LESIONS OF THE BRAIN

Masses within or around the brain may cause a wide range of signs and symptoms. These depend not only on the location and size of the mass, but on the rate of growth. For example, a small mass in a critical (eloquent) location, such as the brainstem, may cause symptoms earlier than a huge but slowly growing mass in a less eloquent location, such as the frontal lobe. Intracranial masses may cause increased intracranial pressure and headache; focal neurologic deficits from compression of brain tissue or nerves; ischemia; obstruction to CSF flow resulting in hydrocephalus; and seizures.

Because many of these clinical manifestations are nonspecific, imaging is important in detecting and characterizing intracranial masses. MRI is the most sensitive imaging modality for many of these processes, although CT is frequently adequate. Intravenous contrast material administration is often helpful. Because of the added expense, risk, and time that accompany administration, guidelines are usually used to select those patients who should receive such contrast injections. Generally accepted indications include suspected metastases, known primary tumor, and newly detected brain masses. Some tumors, such as meningiomas, are dramatically more conspicuous with contrast agent administration.

Neoplasms of the brain are discussed in

this chapter. The list for differential diagnosis of a mass within the brain, however, is long. Infection, hematoma, giant aneurysm, and some uncommon congenital or inflammatory disorders may initially be detected as masses within the brain and hence may be confused with tumor. Infarction and hematoma may occasionally simulate the imaging appearance of an aggressive mass lesion. The presence of ring enhancement may contribute to this confusion. Table 4–1 lists some of the conditions that may appear as ring-enhancing masses of the brain.

CLASSIFICATION OF BRAIN NEOPLASMS

Neoplasms of the brain and its coverings include various tumor types and cells of origin. Occasionally, classification is difficult. To provide order, efficient and descriptive classification schemes may be of assistance. The World Health Organization (WHO) scheme is widely employed. Tumors of glial origin are conveniently considered as a group. These include tumors derived from astrocytes (astrocytoma), oligodendrocytes (oligodendroglioma), and the ependyma that lines the ventricular system (ependymoma). Tumors of choroid plexus origin (choroid plexus papilloma and carcinoma) are also in this group.

Nonglial tumors of the brain originate

TABLE 4–1. **Differential Diagnosis of Ring-enhancing Masses in the Brain**

Primary brain neoplasm
Metastatic neoplasm
Abscess
Subacute infarction
Resolving hematoma
Thrombosed aneurysm or AVM
Multiple sclerosis plaque (on MRI)
Radiation necrosis

from the other types of tissue that are present within the confines of the calvarium. Tumors of neuronal origin are uncommon. Tumors arising from the meninges, in contrast, are very common, particularly meningiomas. Primitive embryonic cells of the brain are the presumed origin of the tumors termed *medulloblastoma* and *primitive neuroectodermal tumor* (PNET). Hematopoietic tumors include lymphoma, leukemia, and plasmacytoma. Several types of germ cell tumors occur, with the pineal region a common but not exclusive location. Schwannomas (neuromas) arise from the third through twelfth cranial nerves (most frequently the eighth). The second cranial nerve, which is histologically an extension of the brain and is lined by meninges, gives rise to optic gliomas and meningiomas. Several neoplasms originate in or around the pituitary gland, especially adenomas and craniopharyngiomas. Metastatic spread is a major source of neoplasms of the brain, meninges, and skull.

A brief discussion of lytic skull processes is included at the end of this chapter. Although extracranial head and neck tumors are not within the scope of this book, the possibility of direct extension of such tumors into or through the skull must be considered.

BRAIN TUMORS OF GLIAL-CELL ORIGIN

Most glial tumors are poorly marginated neoplasms that infiltrate into the surrounding brain. Complete resection is usually difficult, and recurrence is common, even with low-grade tumors. Although extracranial spread is rare, glial neoplasms are not truly benign because of their tendency to infiltrate through the adjacent white matter. Pilocytic astrocytoma (WHO grade I) is an exception, and the patient has a relatively good prognosis.

Astrocytoma

Astrocytomas in the past have been graded on a scale from 1 to 4 (Kernohan system); more recently, a three-grade system (WHO system) has been employed. Grade II, or low grade, in the WHO system, includes Kernohan grades 1 and 2; grade III is anaplastic astrocytoma, and grade IV is glioblastoma multiforme.

Glioblastoma multiforme is a highly aggressive astrocytoma with a poor prognosis. It accounts for about 50 percent of all astrocytomas, making it the most common primary intracranial CNS tumor until recently. (Primary lymphoma of the brain, previously rare, is becoming relatively common.) Necrosis and neovascular proliferation are its pathologic hallmarks. Areas of central necrosis are therefore common. Extensive surrounding vasogenic edema and significant mass effect are often present. The appearance on CT and MRI reflects these characteristics (Fig. 4–1). Attenuation (on CT) or signal intensity (on MRI) is often heterogeneous. Areas of necrosis are seen as fluid-like regions, although the margins of the fluid space are seldom smooth as in a cyst. The apparent outer margin of the tumor is irregular. The margins observed by CT or MRI do not represent the full extent of tumor cells, because infiltration is the rule. Hemorrhage may be present. Surrounding vasogenic edema is readily observed on CT or MRI.

Enhancement varies from intense to patchy, and necrotic areas do not enhance. Enhancement reflects breakdown of the blood-brain barrier, and the infiltrating edges of the tumor that do not produce breakdown of the blood-brain barrier do not enhance. Calcification is uncommon. Extension through white matter tracts may in-

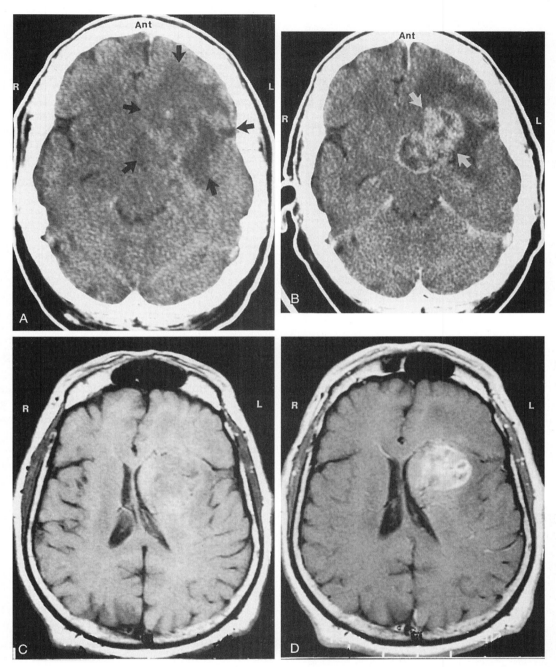

Figure 4–1. Glioblastoma multiforme. *(A)* CT scan before contrast administration shows an irregular area of low density in the left frontal and temporal lobes *(arrows)*. *(B)* After intravenous contrast administration, there is peripheral, nodular enhancement visible on CT *(arrows)*. *(C)* MRI (axial T1WI) demonstrates an ill-defined low signal intensity in the region of the tumor. *(D)* Axial post-gadolinium T1WI from MRI demonstrates a very inhomogeneous enhancement pattern, as well as mass effect and shift of the midline to the right.

Illustration continued on following page

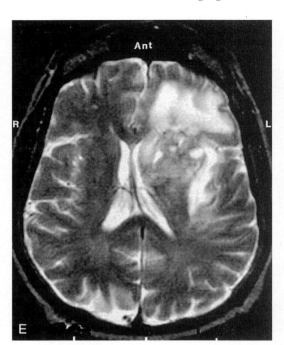

Figure 4–1 *Continued (E)* Axial T2WI also demonstrates a heterogeneous appearance of the tumor, with cystic (necrotic) areas and vasogenic edema. (From Mettler F: Essentials of Radiology. Philadelphia, WB Saunders, 1995, pp 30–31.)

volve the corpus callosum. *Butterfly glioma* is a term that is occasionally used to describe a tumor that has crossed the corpus callosum and has visible adjacent tumor bulk in both hemispheres (Fig. 4–2). There may be a lack of correlation between imaging and histologic features. Therefore, CT or MRI features can imply aggressiveness but are not completely reliable for grading purposes.

Less aggressive astrocytomas may appear less necrotic and cause less edema (Fig. 4–3). Contrast enhancement is usually present. Low-grade astrocytomas can be difficult to identify on scans, especially CT, if there is little edema and no abnormal enhancement.

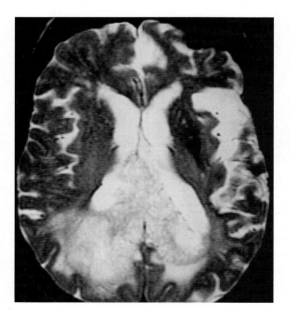

Figure 4–2. Butterfly glioma. MRI (axial T2WI) of a high-grade astrocytoma shows high signal intensity involving the splenium of the corpus callosum and both parietal lobes, with some adjacent vasogenic edema.

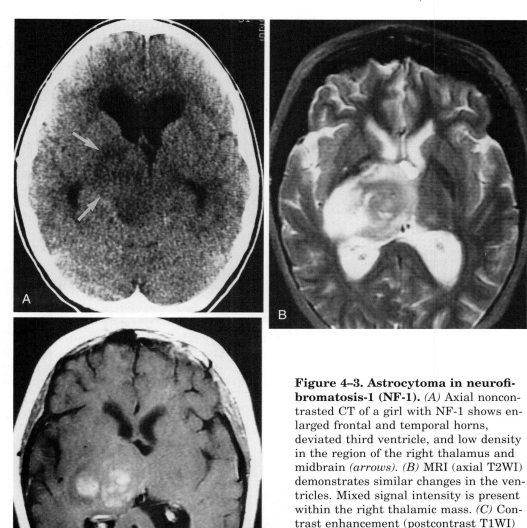

Figure 4–3. Astrocytoma in neurofibromatosis-1 (NF-1). *(A)* Axial noncontrasted CT of a girl with NF-1 shows enlarged frontal and temporal horns, deviated third ventricle, and low density in the region of the right thalamus and midbrain *(arrows)*. *(B)* MRI (axial T2WI) demonstrates similar changes in the ventricles. Mixed signal intensity is present within the right thalamic mass. *(C)* Contrast enhancement (postcontrast T1WI) is inhomogeneous.

Time to recurrence of lower-grade astrocytomas is longer with treatment. The main portion of an astrocytoma is usually of lower attenuation than brain on CT and of high signal intensity on T2-weighted MRI.

Astrocytomas can occur throughout the brain. In children they are common in the cerebellar hemispheres (Fig. 4–4). Brainstem gliomas are usually low grade and often exhibit little to no contrast enhancement (Fig. 4–5). They can extend beyond the brainstem into the upper cervical spinal cord or the cerebellar hemispheres, and they may be exophytic.

Oligodendroglioma

Oligodendrogliomas arise from oligodendrocytes, although there is often a mixed astrocytic component. They constitute only 5 to 10 percent of all gliomas and are associated with a similar infiltrative nature. Distinction from astrocytoma is difficult on scans. Calcification in oligodendrogliomas is fairly common (Fig. 4–6), whereas astrocyto-

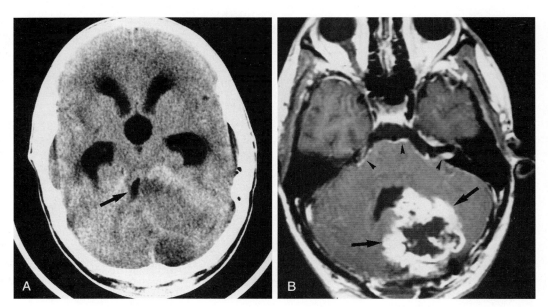

Figure 4–4. Cerebellar astrocytoma with recurrence and subarachnoid spread. *(A)* Initial CT reveals low-density left cerebellar hemisphere mass. The fourth ventricle *(arrow)* is deviated and compressed. The third and lateral ventricles are enlarged. *(B)* Axial T1-weighted MRI 1 year later shows persistent enhancement at the site of the tumor and surgical resection *(arrows),* and scattered areas of leptomeningeal enhancement from spread through the subarachnoid space *(arrowheads).*

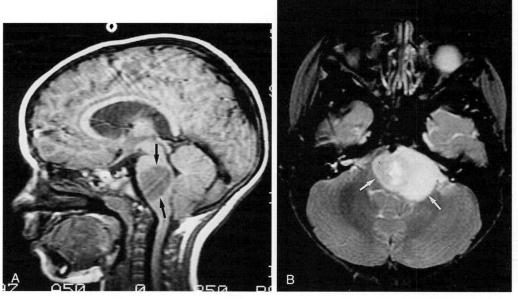

Figure 4–5. Brainstem glioma. MRI of a 5-year-old girl who presented because of difficulty walking. *(A)* The mass expands the pons and has low signal intensity on the sagittal T1WI *(arrows).* *(B)* It has high signal intensity on the T2WI *(arrows).* The fourth ventricle is narrowed, and mild hydrocephalus is present. Only a small area within the tumor showed contrast enhancement.

mas are less often calcified. Because astrocytomas are more common overall, however, calcification in a mass is not specific for tumor type.

Ependymoma

Ependymomas arise from the ependymal lining of the ventricular system. They are common in children, especially in the fourth ventricle (Fig. 4–7). As they fill the fourth ventricle, they can squeeze through the foramina of Luschka and Magendie and lead to subarachnoid spread. Enhancement is variable, although some generally occurs. Because of the tendency for CSF spread of tumor cells, it is usually necessary to evaluate the spine with contrast-enhanced MRI when fourth ventricle ependymomas are initially diagnosed.

Choroid Plexus Tumors

Choroid plexus tumors can be benign (papillomas) or malignant (carcinomas, which are rare). In children they most commonly occur

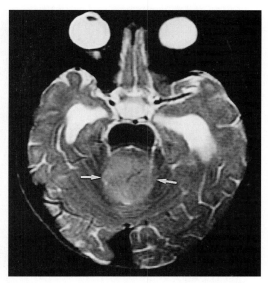

Figure 4–7. Ependymoma. MRI (axial T2WI) of a 1-year-old girl discloses a mass *(arrows)* filling and enlarging the fourth ventricle. Enlarged temporal horns of the lateral ventricles are visible, indicating that obstructive hydrocephalus is present.

in the lateral ventricles, but in adults they are most commonly found in the fourth ventricle. Intense contrast enhancement is nearly always present. Overproduction of CSF or obstruction of the ventricular system may lead to hydrocephalus (Fig. 4–8).

BRAIN TUMORS OF NON–GLIAL-CELL ORIGIN

Medulloblastoma and PNET

Medulloblastoma is an older term for a tumor of small, round cells that occurs in the posterior fossa. *Primitive neuroectodermal tumor* (PNET) is a term for small, round-cell tumors that occur throughout the brain (and elsewhere), and the term is preferred by some for posterior fossa tumors (medulloblastomas) as well. Because of the lower water content than in other tumors (high nuclear-to-cytoplasmic ratio), these tumors often have somewhat higher attenuation than normal brain tissue on CT (Fig. 4–9). The signal intensity on T2-weighted MRI

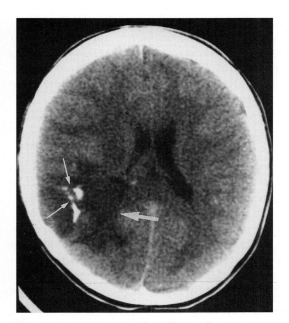

Figure 4–6. Oligodendroglioma in a nonenhanced CT scan of a young woman. Low density *(large arrow)* and focal areas of irregular calcification *(small arrows)* are present. As is often the case with oligodendroglioma, there was a mixed astrocytic component as well.

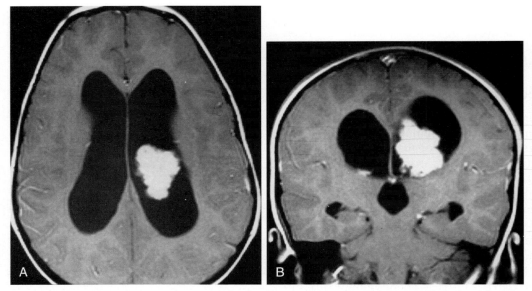

Figure 4–8. Choroid plexus papilloma. Contrast-enhanced MRI of a 3-year-old boy with hydrocephalus without evidence of obstruction. *(A)* Axial and *(B)* coronal T1WI demonstrate a somewhat lobulated, intensely enhancing mass within the body of the left lateral ventricle. The ventricles are dilated. (Courtesy of Dr. M. Gutíerrez.)

also may not be as high as is typically observed with astrocytomas, but this is variable. Enhancement is common, and cyst formation and calcification can occur. Near the fourth ventricle, the medullary velum is a common site of origin. However, a smaller percentage of medulloblastomas, particularly in older children and adults, can originate in the cerebellar hemispheres. A high percentage of medulloblastomas occur in childhood, but they can also occur in young adults.

Lymphoma

Lymphoma uncommonly spreads to the brain from elsewhere in the body. Historically, primary lymphoma of the brain was rare. More recently, however, because of its association with immunocompromised patients, lymphoma of the brain is becoming increasingly common and will likely overtake astrocytoma as the most common primary brain neoplasm (Fig. 4–10).

Lymphoma is often hyperdense compared with brain on CT. MRI signal intensity is somewhat variable. Deep cerebral locations are common, but other locations can also occur. Some contrast enhancement is usu-

ally present and can be ring-like or diffuse. In the immunocompromised patient, lymphoma can occasionally be difficult to differentiate from *Toxoplasma* abscess. Although some imaging features are more common in lymphoma than in toxoplasmosis, there is significant overlap, and follow-up examinations after empiric therapy for toxoplasmosis are often the most helpful.

Hemangioblastoma

Hemangioblastoma is an uncommon and extremely vascular tumor of the CNS. In about two thirds of cases, patients present with a tumor nodule along the wall of a cyst, whereas in the remaining one third the tumors are solid. The tumor shows intense contrast enhancement on CT or MRI. Angiography demonstrates a dense tumor blush. The cerebellum is the most common location (Fig. 4–11). Hemangioblastomas also occur less commonly in other locations in the brain and in the spinal cord. About one sixth of patients with hemangioblastoma have von Hippel-Lindau disease, a neurocutaneous syndrome (see Chapter 9). The differential diagnosis of a cyst with an en-

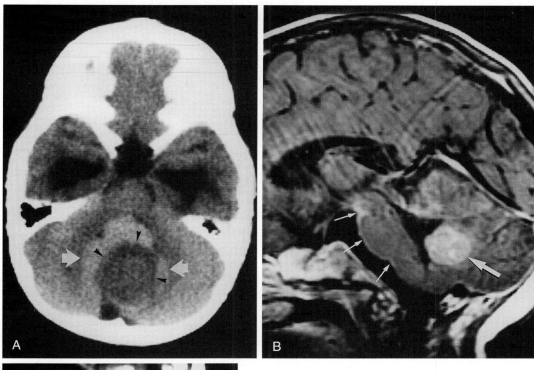

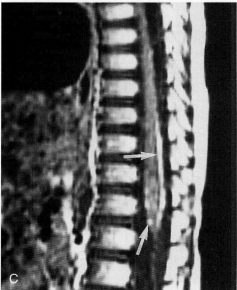

Figure 4–9. Medulloblastoma with CSF spread. *(A)* Initial nonenhanced CT scan reveals a large, dense posterior fossa mass *(arrows)* with a low-density cystic component *(arrowheads)*. The tumor itself is denser than normal brain. *(B, C)* Follow-up MRI scan a year later shows recurrence and extensive spread through the subarachnoid space. *(B)* Sagittal post-gadolinium T1WI of the brain demonstrates an enhancing mass dorsal to the fourth ventricle *(large arrow)* and superficial enhancement along the surface of the brainstem and cerebellum *(small arrows)*. (This "sugar-coating" appearance is sometimes referred to as "zuckerguss.") *(C)* Sagittal post-gadolinium T1WI of the spine also demonstrates enhancing leptomeningeal metastases along the surface of the distal spinal cord *(arrows)*.

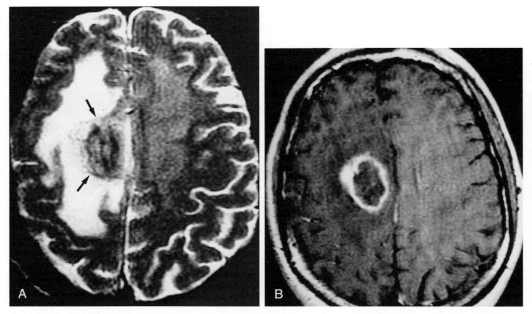

Figure 4–10. Lymphoma. MRI of a young man with AIDS. *(A)* Axial T2WI shows a heterogeneous mass in the right cerebral hemisphere with <u>extensive surrounding vasogenic edema.</u> *(B)* Following gadolinium administration (T1WI), there is irregular peripheral enhancement. Toxoplasmosis is the primary differential consideration, but the lesion grew despite empiric therapy for toxoplasmosis. Biopsy was then performed and confirmed the diagnosis of primary brain lymphoma.

hancing mural nodule includes cystic astrocytoma, metastasis, and hemangioblastoma.

Neuronal-origin Tumors

Tumors of neuronal origin are uncommon in the CNS. Ganglioglioma is a low-grade neoplasm that usually occurs in teenagers or young adults (Fig. 4–12). The temporal lobe is a common location. Enhancement is variable. Prominent cystic components are often present, and calcification is common. Central neurocytoma is an uncommon neoplasm, typically manifesting as an intraventricular hemorrhagic mass.

Germ-cell Tumors

Several types of germ-cell origin neoplasms occur around the CNS. Lipomas of the CNS are probably developmental anomalies of the subarachnoid space (meninx primitiva). (See Chapter 9 regarding lipomas of the corpus callosum.) The interhemispheric fissure, suprasellar cistern, quadrigeminal cistern, and cerebellopontine angle are common locations. Intracranial lipomas have a tendency to occur in and around the midline. CT and MRI show the typical imaging appearance of fat (see Fig. 9–7). Calcification is frequently present.

Epidermoid tumors or cysts are composed of epithelial debris within a squamous epithelial–lined cyst. They are probably the result of inclusions of ectodermal epithelial elements during development of the brain. The outer surface is irregular, and a characteristic frond-like appearance is observed if a cisternogram is obtained. Epidermoid tumors are of low density on CT and usually have signal intensity very close to that of CSF on MRI. Subtle differences from CSF signal intensity are often observed on the intermediate-weighted images. They rarely demonstrate contrast enhancement. The cerebellopontine angle is the most common location for these tumors (Fig. 4–13). Typically, they occur in off-midline sites. Epidermoid tumors can also arise in the skull (see Table 4–4).

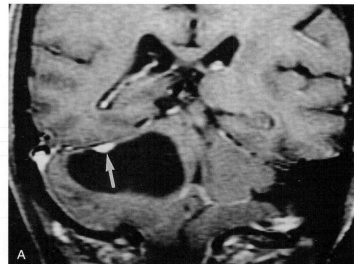

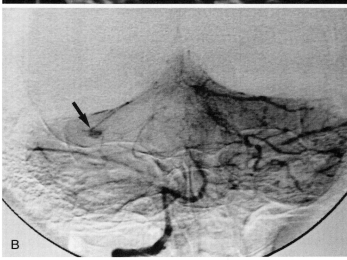

Figure 4–11. Hemangioblastoma. *(A)* MRI (coronal T1WI) obtained after gadolinium contrast administration shows a large right cerebellar hemisphere cyst and an enhancing nodule *(arrow)* along the superior margin. *(B)* Arteriogram with right vertebral artery injection demonstrates a vascular blush in the area of the nodule *(arrow)*.

Unlike epidermoid tumors, dermoid tumors tend to lie near the midline. They contain dermal appendages, such as hair and sebaceous and sweat glands, as well as an epithelial lining. They also do not enhance. Fat attenuation or signal intensity is often observed on CT or MRI, respectively. Dermoids can rupture into the subarachnoid space or ventricular system and cause an inflammatory meningitis or ventriculitis (Fig. 4–14).

Teratomas have elements of more than one germ layer. Several varieties occur in the CNS. Little enhancement usually occurs. Fat and calcification are common, and the imaging appearance is heterogeneous. The pineal region is the most common location. Germinomas are more common and also occur most often in the pineal region (Fig. 4–15).

NEOPLASMS OF THE MENINGES

Meningioma

Meningioma is one of the more common intracranial neoplasms. It is the most common non-glial primary brain tumor and represents 15 to 20 percent of all primary brain tumors. Most of these tumors of meningothelial origin are benign. Atypical or malignant types are uncommon. They usually grow slowly and sometimes reach a large size before coming to clinical attention.

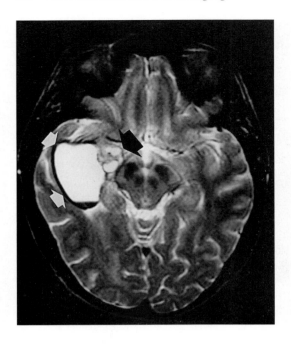

Figure 4–12. Ganglioglioma. Axial MRI (T2WI) of a young woman with a medial, right temporal lobe mass. Several small cysts *(black arrow)* and a single large cyst *(white arrows)* are present. There has been some hemorrhage within the large cyst.

They present most often in middle age, with predominance in females. Progesterone receptors are frequently demonstrated in meningiomas, as are abnormalities of chromosome 22. The cerebral convexities, falx cerebri, and sphenoid wing are common locations, but they can appear in any site where meningeal tissue is present. Ninety percent are supratentorial. The tumors are frequently denser than normal brain, and calcification is common. They are often quite vascular. Most meningiomas are fed by branches of the external carotid artery, but internal carotid artery branches can be recruited by larger tumors as well as tumors located along the tentorium.

Imaging features of meningiomas reflect these characteristics (Figs. 4–16, 4–17). Extra-axial masses are adjacent to the dura mater, usually with a rounded or hemispheric shape. A variant known as en plaque meningioma is more flat and can appear as sheet-like thickening along the dura. Larger tumors displace underlying brain, with buckling of the cortex. Vasogenic edema is often present in the affected areas of the underlying brain and is easily seen on CT and MRI. The tumors usually have higher attenuation than brain on CT. Signal intensity is somewhat variable on MRI, but the typical meningioma is nearly isointense with brain on all pulse sequences. Small meningiomas can, therefore, be difficult to identify without contrast material administration. Nearly all meningiomas show intense contrast enhancement. A dural tail of enhancement extending into the contiguous dura mater is often present (see Fig. 4–16), but this appearance is not specific for meningioma. Calcifications are occasionally observed on CT. Cyst formation is less common.

Angiography shows an early, dense, and prolonged vascular blush (see Fig. 4–17). The blush often occurs in a sunburst pattern that reflects the dural vascular supply radiating outward from a central pedicle. In addition to its diagnostic value, angiography can be helpful for presurgical planning. Preoperative percutaneous intravascular embolization of meningiomas may be performed to aid in control of surgical bleeding. An osteoblastic reaction (hyperostosis) is often noted in the adjacent bone and can be seen on CT or plain films of the skull.

Hemangiopericytoma

Hemangiopericytoma is an uncommon neoplasm that can originate in the meninges

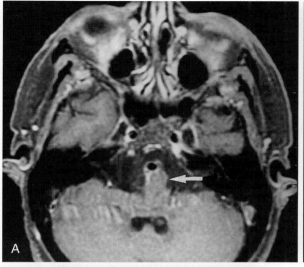

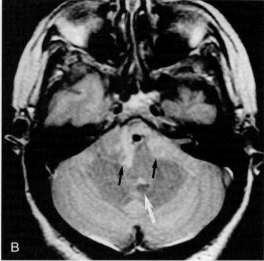

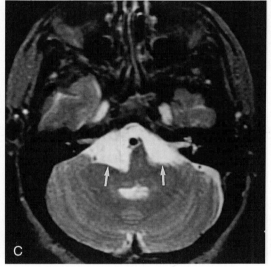

Figure 4–13. Cerebellopontine angle epidermoid. MRI of a woman with multiple cranial nerve deficits. *(A)* Axial T1WI (after gadolinium administration) shows a narrowed, distorted brainstem *(arrow)*. Tissue anterior and lateral to the brainstem has low signal intensity, which is similar to CSF. There is no contrast enhancement of this tissue. *(B)* On the intermediate-weighted axial image (long TR/short TE), the epidermoid tumor *(black arrows)* has more heterogeneous signal intensity and is slightly brighter than CSF in the fourth ventricle *(white arrow)*. *(C)* Signal intensity on the axial T2WI (long TR/long TE) of the epidermoid is bright *(arrows),* which is again similar to CSF.

and may simulate closely the appearance of meningioma. The tumors derive from contractile cells (pericytes) that occur around capillaries, rather than from the meningothelial arachnoid cap cell. Many "angioblastic" meningiomas, a subtype described in the past, are probably hemangiopericytomas. They are highly vascular and more aggressive in behavior than typical meningiomas.

METASTATIC NEOPLASMS

Hematogenous Metastasis

Hematogenous spread of neoplasm to the brain is very common. Metastases account for up to one third of all brain tumors. In addition to evaluation of the symptomatic patient with a known primary neoplasm, imaging of the brain for metastases is sometimes performed as part of staging and is done prior to therapy. Therapy of metastases to the brain can include radiation, chemotherapy for some tumors, and, in selected cases, surgical resection of solitary metastases.

Lung and breast carcinoma commonly spread to the brain, followed by melanoma and gastrointestinal and genitourinary tumors. A wide range of other neoplasms can also metastasize to the brain. Melanoma, choriocarcinoma, and renal cell carcinoma

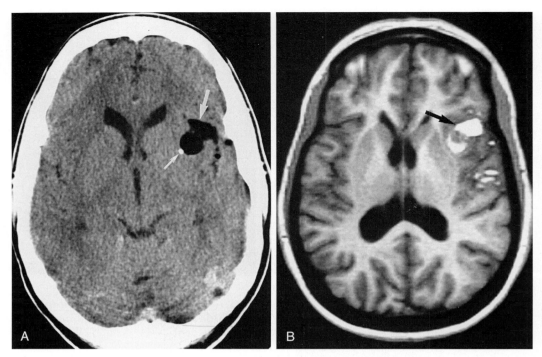

Figure 4–14. Dermoid cyst. *(A)* CT of a woman with severe headache discloses a mass in the left sylvian fissure region with fat attenuation *(large arrow)* and a small focus of calcification *(small arrow).* Separate areas of low density are present in the subarachnoid space of the sylvian fissure. *(B)* Axial MRI (T1WI) also demonstrates the presence of fat (high signal intensity) within the dermoid cyst *(arrow),* which had ruptured, and fat elsewhere in the subarachnoid space from rupture.

are particularly prone to hemorrhagic metastases (see Fig. 6–15). Occasionally a tumor can present as a hemorrhage and initially can be obscured by the blood. Diagnosis in these cases can be difficult, and repeat examination after resolution of the hemorrhage may be necessary. Detection of additional masses, especially with enhancement, can suggest the presence of metastases.

Metastases can occur in a variety of locations but are often found at the gray-white matter junction. Surrounding vasogenic edema is often present. Attenuation on CT or signal intensity on MRI can vary, but metastases often have a higher water content than brain (Fig. 4–18). Hemorrhage within a tumor can alter its appearance. The appearance of intracranial hemorrhage is discussed in Chapter 6. It should be noted that hemorrhage within neoplasms can sometimes be complex or atypical compared with hemorrhage from other sources. Be-

cause an abnormal blood-brain barrier is present, metastases usually demonstrate contrast enhancement. If there is strong suspicion of metastases, intravenous contrast material should be administered. MRI is more sensitive than CT for small metastases.

Other Types of Metastatic Spread

Because the brain does not have a lymphatic system like other organs, lymphatic spread is not seen. However, other pathways of tumor spread to and within the CNS should be recognized. Some tumors, especially squamous cell carcinoma of the head and adenoid cystic carcinoma, have a propensity to extend along peripheral nerves. These tumors can even extend intracranially by this perineural route. For example, skin cancers or salivary gland cancers can extend along branches of the fifth cranial nerve through the skull base. The

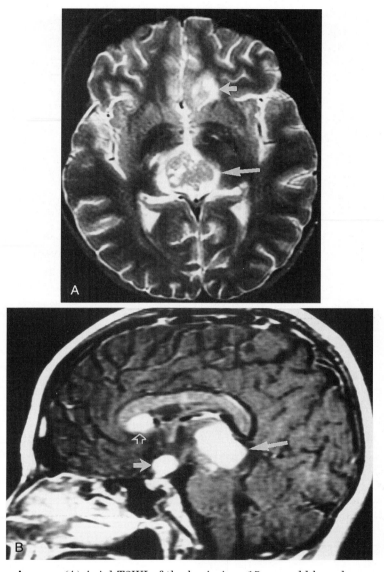

Figure 4–15. Germinoma. *(A)* Axial T2WI of the brain in a 15-year-old boy shows a pineal region mass *(long arrow)* with slightly higher signal intensity than brain and smaller areas of very high signal intensity. Abnormal signal intensity is also present near the tip of the left frontal horn *(short arrow)*. *(B)* On the sagittal post-gadolinium T1WI, there is intense contrast enhancement of the pineal region mass *(long arrow)*. Two other enhancing masses are present, one in the suprasellar cistern *(short solid arrow)* and the other near the rostrum of the corpus callosum *(short open arrow)*.

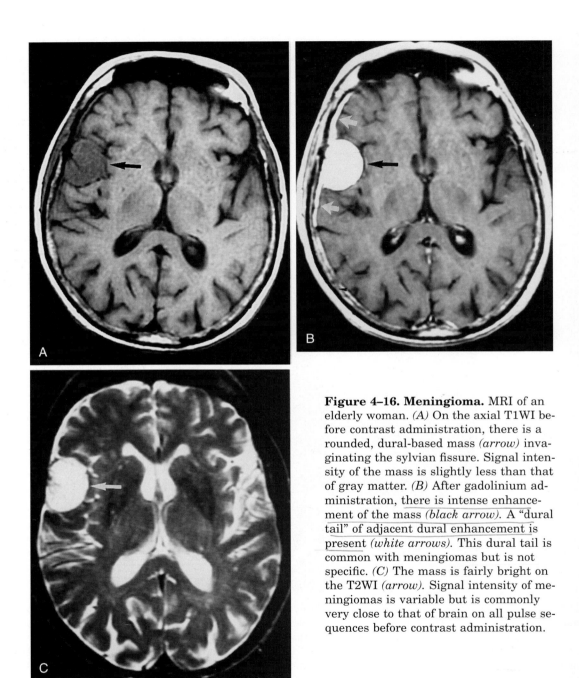

Figure 4–16. Meningioma. MRI of an elderly woman. *(A)* On the axial T1WI before contrast administration, there is a rounded, dural-based mass *(arrow)* invaginating the sylvian fissure. Signal intensity of the mass is slightly less than that of gray matter. *(B)* After gadolinium administration, there is intense enhancement of the mass *(black arrow)*. A "dural tail" of adjacent dural enhancement is present *(white arrows)*. This dural tail is common with meningiomas but is not specific. *(C)* The mass is fairly bright on the T2WI *(arrow)*. Signal intensity of meningiomas is variable but is commonly very close to that of brain on all pulse sequences before contrast administration.

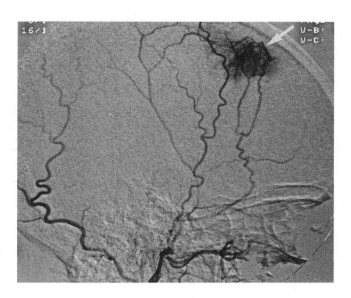

Figure 4–17. Meningioma. Lateral projection of arteriogram (external carotid artery injection) performed on a 50-year-old woman shows middle meningeal artery branches supplying a mass with prominent vascular blush *(arrow)*. Dense blush persisted well into the venous phase.

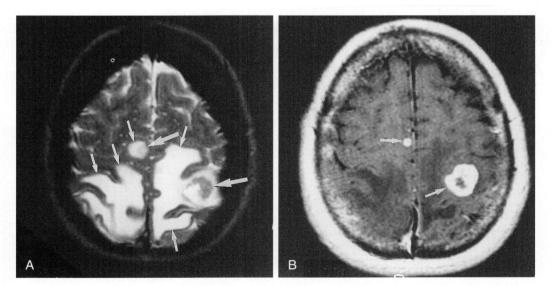

Figure 4–18. Metastases to the brain. MRI of the brain in a woman with known lung cancer. *(A)* Axial T2WI shows high signal intensity from vasogenic edema *(small arrows)*, and lower signal intensity from the masses themselves *(large arrows)*. *(B)* Post-gadolinium T1WI reveals ring-like enhancement of a small, right posterior, frontal lobe metastasis *(small arrow)* and dense enhancement of a larger lesion on the patient's left *(large arrow)* with probable central necrosis. Edema is darker on the T1WI. A larger area of edema on the right is from a third lesion seen on more inferior slices.

foramina in the skull base, such as the foramen ovale, can be enlarged in these cases, and abnormal enhancement is usually present.

Neoplasms can also spread through the CSF to other intracranial or intraspinal locations. Meningeal spread of tumor is best visualized with contrast-enhanced MRI. It appears as nodular or sheet-like areas of enhancement on T1-weighted images. Primary brain tumors can spread in this manner (see Figs. 4–4, 4–9), and extracranial metastatic disease to the meninges also occurs (see Fig. 12–21).

SELLAR REGION MASSES

Patients with masses in and around the sella turcica can present with endocrine symptoms, compression of the optic chiasm or cranial nerves passing through the cavernous sinus, or mass effect on the brain itself. CSF obstruction at the level of the third ventricle uncommonly results from large suprasellar masses. Endocrinologic symptoms result from excessive secretion of anterior pituitary hormones from adenomas or from compressive effects of masses (in-

cluding hormonally-inactive adenomas) on the pituitary gland or hypothalamus. Because of multiplanar capability, lack of artifact from bone at the skull base, and sensitivity to contrast material, MRI is the best imaging test for most sellar region masses.

Pituitary Adenomas

Pituitary adenomas are common and histologically benign neoplasms. Microadenomas are defined as those less than 1 cm in diameter. They come to clinical attention because of hypersecretion syndromes such as galactorrhea/amenorrhea (from hyperprolactinemia), Cushing's syndrome (from elevated ACTH), and acromegaly (from elevated growth hormone). They cause little or no deformity in the contour of the pituitary gland. Although signal intensity of microadenomas can differ from that of normal pituitary gland, the most sensitive imaging feature is delayed gadolinium enhancement of a microadenoma as compared with the normal gland. For this reason, dynamic MRI sequences using rapid acquisition following intravenous contrast administration are often helpful (Fig. 4–19). Because asymptomatic, nonfunctional microadenomas are fairly common in the general popu-

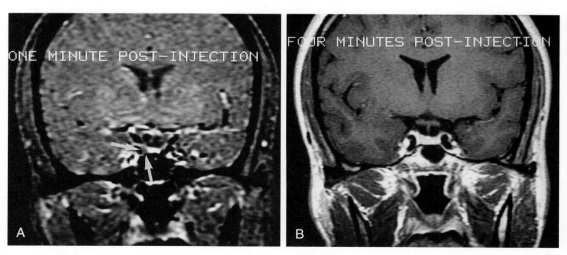

Figure 4–19. Pituitary microadenoma. *(A)* Coronal T1WI from dynamic MRI (i.e., rapid acquisition of images after contrast administration) in a 36-year-old woman with elevated prolactin. A small, round area in the right side of the pituitary gland shows less enhancement than the rest of the gland 1 minute after injection *(arrows)*. *(B)* At an identical level 4 minutes after injection, the area appears more normal. Delayed enhancement relative to normal pituitary tissue is typical of microadenomas.

lation, correlation with endocrine study results is necessary in interpreting the significance of incidentally detected microadenomas.

Adenomas larger than 1 cm in diameter are arbitrarily termed *macroadenomas.* Patients are more likely to present because of mass effect on cranial nerves or the brain. Bitemporal hemianopsia from compression of the optic chiasm is a classic presentation. The tumors can grow superiorly through the diaphragma sellae into the suprasellar cistern, inferiorly into the sphenoid sinus, or laterally into the cavernous sinus. The intracavernous internal carotid artery can be encased by tumor. Delineating the extent of such growth is important in presurgical planning.

Spontaneous hemorrhage within pituitary adenomas is common and often asymptomatic. *Pituitary apoplexy* is a term that is most properly applied to the clinical syndrome of sudden, severe headache, visual loss, and ophthalmoplegia resulting from hemorrhage into a macroadenoma. Pituitary apoplexy is a clinical emergency and an indication for immediate imaging. Macroadenomas are readily identified on MRI as masses originating in the sella (Fig. 4–20).

Other Pituitary Region Masses

Craniopharyngioma is a tumor of neuroepithelial origin. Cystic components and calcification are very common. The peak age of presentation is in childhood and adolescence, but there is a second peak (bimodal) later in life. Tumors can arise above or within the sella. Signal intensity of the fluid component on MRI varies. The solid component of the tumor usually enhances. CT can be a useful supplemental test to identify calcification (Fig. 4–21).

Other less common intrasellar masses also occur. Rathke's cleft cysts result from remnants of Rathke's pouch. They appear as simple cysts within or above the pituitary gland. Although the wall may enhance, there is no nodular neoplastic component. Pituitary carcinomas and pituitary abscesses are rare. Metastases to the pituitary gland have been reported.

Gliomas may arise from the optic nerves or occur more posteriorly along the optic pathways. Gliomas of the optic chiasm may appear as suprasellar masses. Most optic gliomas are low-grade neoplasms, and enhancement is variable. There is an increased incidence in neurofibromatosis-1 (see Chapter 9).

Aneurysms of the cavernous sinus segment of the internal carotid artery are uncommon but important sources of intrasellar masses. Patients may present because of cranial nerve palsies (Fig. 4–22). Meningiomas of the tuberculum sellae may be difficult to distinguish from adenomas. Their appearance is similar to that of meningio-

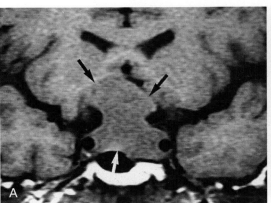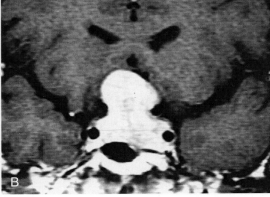

Figure 4–20. Pituitary macroadenoma. MRI (coronal T1WI) before *(A)* and after *(B)* gadolinium contrast administration. A dumbbell-shaped mass *(arrows)* arises from the sella turcica and extends into the suprasellar cistern nearly to the hypothalamus. The patient had severe visual loss. The tumor is slightly hypointense relative to brain before contrast administration and enhances intensely.

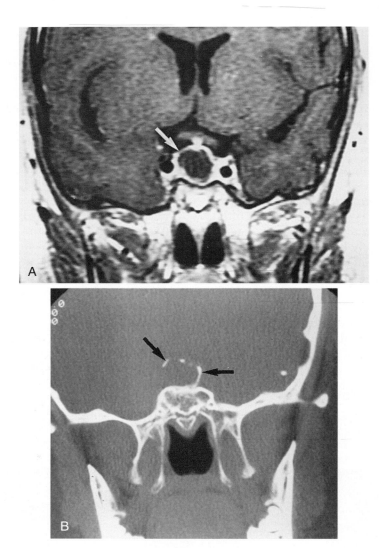

Figure 4–21. Craniopharyngioma. *(A)* Coronal MRI of a 19-year-old woman with primary amenor-rhea and visual field defect. T1WI after contrast administration shows a sellar and suprasellar cystic mass *(arrow)*. There is low signal intensity of fluid within the enhancing rim. *(B)* Coronal CT (bone window) reveals calcification within the rim *(arrows)*.

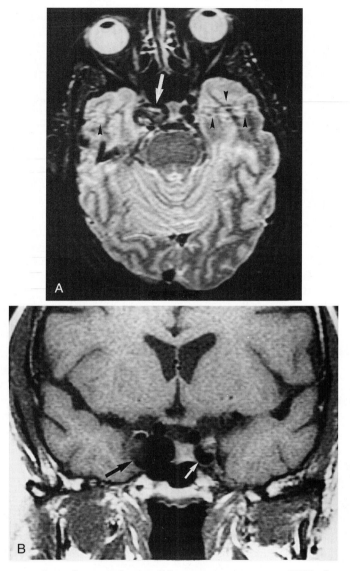

Figure 4–22. Cavernous sinus internal carotid artery aneurysm. MRI of a woman with the complaint of double vision. *(A)* Axial T2WI shows a rounded area of very heterogeneous signal intensity *(white arrow)* in the right cavernous sinus and a band of flow-related artifact *(arrowheads)* in the phase-encoding direction. Mixed signal intensity within the aneurysm is caused by turbulent flow. *(B)* Coronal T1WI demonstrates a round, dark area of signal void in the aneurysm *(black arrow)* in the right cavernous sinus. Compare this appearance with the normal left side, where the carotid siphon is cut in cross-section *(white arrow).*

TABLE 4–2. **Sellar Region Masses**

Pituitary adenoma
  Microadenoma
  Macroadenoma
Meningioma
Craniopharyngioma
Optic glioma
Hypothalamic glioma
Aneurysm
Germinoma, other germ-cell tumor
Pituitary hyperplasia
Metastasis
Hypophysitis
Histiocytosis
Rathke's cleft cyst
Abscess
Sarcoidosis
Tuberculosis, other basilar cistern
  inflammatory processes

TABLE 4–3. **Cerebellopontine Angle Masses**

Acoustic (vestibular) schwannoma (most
  common)
Meningioma (second most common)
Epidermoid (third most common)
Other cranial nerve schwannoma
Paraganglioma
Astrocytoma (brainstem or cerebellar)
Metastasis
Aneurysm or vascular malformation

mas elsewhere within the cranium. Other masses that can arise in the sellar and parasellar region are listed in Table 4–2.

CEREBELLOPONTINE ANGLE MASSES

Acoustic schwannoma or neuroma is the most common mass of the cerebellopontine angle (CPA). They originate in the internal auditory canal (IAC). Most arise from vestibular divisions of the eighth cranial nerve. MRI is the most sensitive imaging test. Signal intensity is variable before contrast material administration. The rounded mass usually shows considerable enhancement, although necrotic or cystic regions can exist. Larger lesions can compress the brainstem (Fig. 4–23). Bilateral acoustic schwannomas occur in and are diagnostic of neurofibromatosis-2 (see Chapter 9).

Meningiomas are also common masses of the CPA. They demonstrate intense contrast enhancement but do not originate from the IAC. Epidermoid tumors are the third most common CPA mass. They do not enhance,

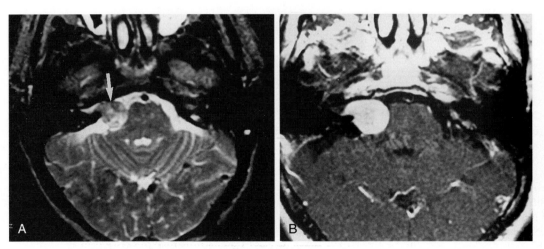

Figure 4–23. Acoustic schwannoma (neuroma). MRI of a 58-year-old man. *(A)* Axial T2WI shows a rounded, mixed-signal-intensity mass *(arrow)* in the right cerebellopontine angle, indenting the brainstem. The internal auditory canal (IAC) is slightly expanded. *(B)* Axial post-contrast T1WI appearance makes it clear that the mass also enhances and involves the medial aspect of the right IAC.

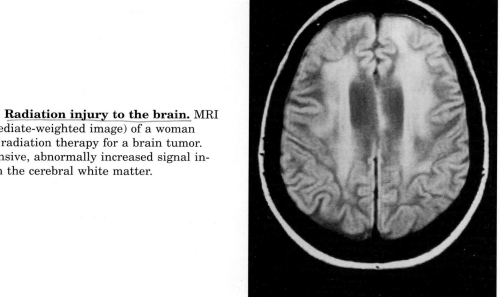

Figure 4–24. Radiation injury to the brain. MRI (axial intermediate-weighted image) of a woman who received radiation therapy for a brain tumor. There is extensive, abnormally increased signal intensity within the cerebral white matter.

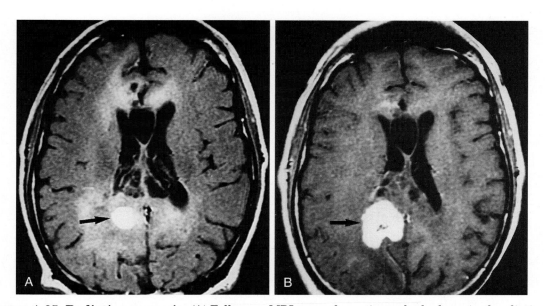

Figure 4–25. Radiation necrosis. *(A)* Follow-up MRI scan of a patient who had received radiation therapy for an oligodendroglioma (post-gadolinium T1WI) demonstrates a right parietal lobe enhancing mass measuring approximately 1 cm in diameter *(arrow)*. (A large cavum septi pellucidi is an incidental finding.) *(B)* Four months later, the mass *(arrow)* had significantly increased in size. The mass was resected and found to represent radiation necrosis.

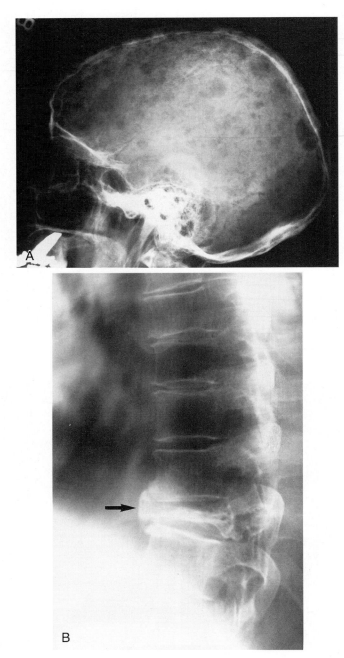

Figure 4–26. Multiple myeloma. *(A)* Lateral skull radiograph demonstrates extensive areas of destruction, sometimes referred to as punched-out lesions, without evidence of surrounding sclerosis. (From Mettler F: Essentials of Radiology. Philadelphia, WB Saunders, 1995, p 16.) *(B)* Lateral thoracic spine radiograph shows loss of bone density and severe compression of one vertebral body *(arrow)*.

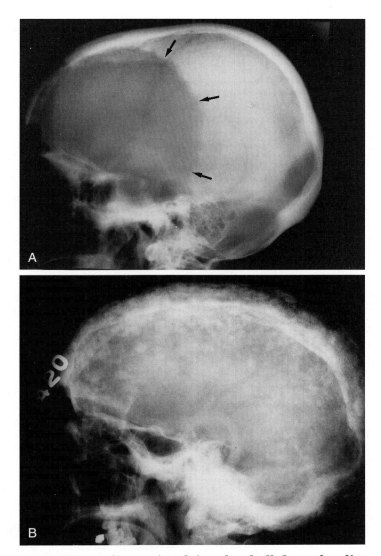

Figure 4–27. Two cases of Paget disease involving the skull (lateral radiographs). *(A)* Large geographic area *(arrows)* of bone loss (osteoporosis circumscripta) without sclerosis (lytic phase). *(B)* Cotton-wool appearance from the sclerotic phase. (From Mettler F: Essentials of Radiology. Philadelphia, WB Saunders, 1995, p 16.)

and they often infiltrate the nearby cisterns (see Fig. 4–13). Other masses that may be observed in this region are listed in Table 4–3.

CONSEQUENCES OF TREATMENT OF BRAIN TUMORS

Imaging studies are often repeated following surgery, chemotherapy, or radiation therapy for brain tumors. New growth at the tumor site and increased contrast enhancement are worrisome and suggest recurrence or growth, although radiation necrosis must also be considered. Delayed radiation necrosis can occur years after therapy and probably results from vascular injury.

Radiation therapy for brain tumors often results in white matter changes, with increased signal intensity on T2-weighted MRI (Fig. 4–24). Radiation necrosis occa-

TABLE 4–4. **Typical Radiographic Features of Common Skull Lesions**

Metastases	Often multiple, ill-defined lytic defects, usually no sclerosis
Myeloma	Often multiple, "punched-out" lytic lesions, no sclerosis
Paget disease (lytic; osteoporosis circumscripta)	Geographic regions of demineralization
Paget disease (reparative phase)	"Cotton-wool" appearance; irregular, dense bone
Epidermoid	Lytic solitary lesion with smooth margin and sclerotic rim
Hemangioma	Lytic solitary lesion with sharp margin, no sclerosis, sometimes a sunburst or soap-bubble appearance
Histiocytosis	Lytic lesion with irregular margin, bevelled edge; no sclerosis initially, but sclerosis may appear with healing
Osteomyelitis	Lytic lesion with permeative appearance, irregular margins, and sclerosis

sionally causes enhancement around a region of central necrosis. This can be very difficult to distinguish from recurrent tumor (Fig. 4–25). Single-photon emission CT (SPECT) studies, positron emission tomography (PET), and MR spectroscopy all have been suggested as tools to distinguish radiation necrosis from viable neoplasm. Radiation therapy also carries a delayed risk of causing meningiomas and sarcomas.

SKULL LESIONS

The differential diagnosis of sclerotic and lytic skull lesions includes both neoplastic

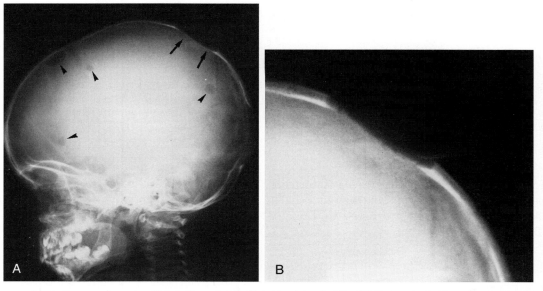

Figure 4–28. Langerhans cell histiocytosis (histiocytosis X). *(A)* Lateral skull radiograph of a 2-year-old child with diabetes insipidus. Multiple, well-defined lytic areas *(arrowheads)* are present in the skull, with no surrounding sclerosis. (From Mettler F: Essentials of Radiology. Philadelphia, WB Saunders, 1995, p 384.) *(B)* Magnified view (region of longer arrows on *A*) of a parietal bone lesion, observed tangentially, shows location within the diploë and a bevelled edge.

and non-neoplastic diseases. A summary of common lesions is presented in Table 4–4.

Metastases to the skull are relatively common. They are often lytic, with ill-defined margins. Multiple myeloma typically produces multiple "punched-out" lesions (Fig. 4–26).

Paget disease (osteitis deformans) is a disorder occurring in middle age, more often in men than in women. Solitary or multiple bones throughout the body are affected, frequently including the skull. An initial lytic phase is followed by a reparative phase, with sclerosis. Well-defined lytic regions in the skull are typical of the first phase (Fig. 4–27A). Sclerosis and a cotton-wool appearance result from later abnormal bone formation (Fig. 4–27B). Softening of the skull base can result in basilar impression.

Langerhans cell histiocytosis includes a spectrum of conditions ranging from eosinophilic granuloma to Hand-Schüller-Christian disease. Skull lesions lack a sclerotic rim, and a bevelled appearance is occasionally observed (Fig. 4–28).

Chapter

5

Ischemia and Related Vascular Diseases of the Brain

Stroke is a major cause of morbidity and mortality, and constitutes the third most common cause of death after heart disease and cancer. Its clinical hallmark is the sudden onset of a focal neurologic deficit. Various treatment options are available. In addition to medical therapy, recent trials of carotid endarterectomy have demonstrated that some patients with carotid atherosclerotic disease may benefit from surgery. Imaging plays a major role in the evaluation of patients with ischemic symptoms, both for the identification of the causes and for guidance of the decision-making process. Although embolic and thrombotic infarctions are very common, other etiologies of ischemia must also be recognized. Conditions presenting primarily with ischemic symptoms are discussed in this chapter, whereas other vascular diseases, especially those presenting primarily with hemorrhage, are discussed in the following chapter.

Medical intervention in acute stroke is currently a subject of intense investigation. Attention has been given both to cytoprotective and thrombolytic strategies in an attempt to protect or rescue areas of the brain at risk. Such approaches require an emphasis on early recognition of symptoms and rapid entry of the patient into the medical system. Imaging of the brain is an integral component of such treatment programs.

ARTERIAL OCCLUSION

The most common etiology of stroke in the adult is occlusion of an artery resulting from either thrombus formation or embolism, with atherosclerosis the most common underlying cause. Carotid artery disease is especially common. The bifurcation of the common carotid artery and origins of the internal and external carotid arteries are frequent locations. Proximal carotid artery disease is readily imaged and is accessible for possible surgical intervention (endarterectomy). The distal internal carotid artery is also a common site for atherosclerosis but is less amenable to imaging and surgical intervention. Intracranial atherosclerosis and vertebral artery disease are common. Ulcerated plaques near the carotid bifurcation are a frequent source of emboli, but the heart must also be considered as a source.

Thrombotic infarctions tend to involve large vascular distributions. Patients may present clinically with premonitory symptoms. Infarctions caused by emboli, however, often involve smaller vessels and show luxury perfusion from collateral circulation more quickly. Embolic infarctions are often distinguished clinically by a deficit that is complete at onset.

Imaging Appearance

CT is usually the first imaging test used to exclude hemorrhage in cases of suspected infarction. CT is often normal in the first few hours of infarction or ischemia, sometimes for up to 24 hours (Fig. 5–1). Subtle effacement of sulci may be an important early clue to infarction. Some of the very earliest signs of middle cerebral or internal carotid artery infarction on CT are (1) loss of the insular stripe of gray matter (loss of gray-white distinction) on the affected side; (2) low attenuation in the ipsilateral caudate head if the perforating arteries are also affected; and (3) a dense (high attenuation) middle cerebral artery, representing clot within the artery (Fig. 5–2). With time, there is increasingly well-defined low attenuation in an area of infarction because of cytotoxic and vasogenic edema. Over several days, there is increasing mass effect from the edema, and large infarctions often manifest significant midline shift or ventricular effacement at this time (see Figs. 5–1, 5–2). Thrombotic infarctions often involve a large

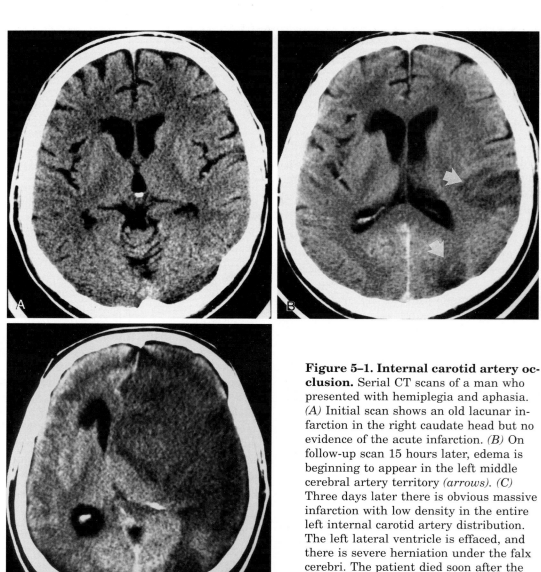

Figure 5–1. Internal carotid artery occlusion. Serial CT scans of a man who presented with hemiplegia and aphasia. *(A)* Initial scan shows an old lacunar infarction in the right caudate head but no evidence of the acute infarction. *(B)* On follow-up scan 15 hours later, edema is beginning to appear in the left middle cerebral artery territory *(arrows)*. *(C)* Three days later there is obvious massive infarction with low density in the entire left internal carotid artery distribution. The left lateral ventricle is effaced, and there is severe herniation under the falx cerebri. The patient died soon after the last scan.

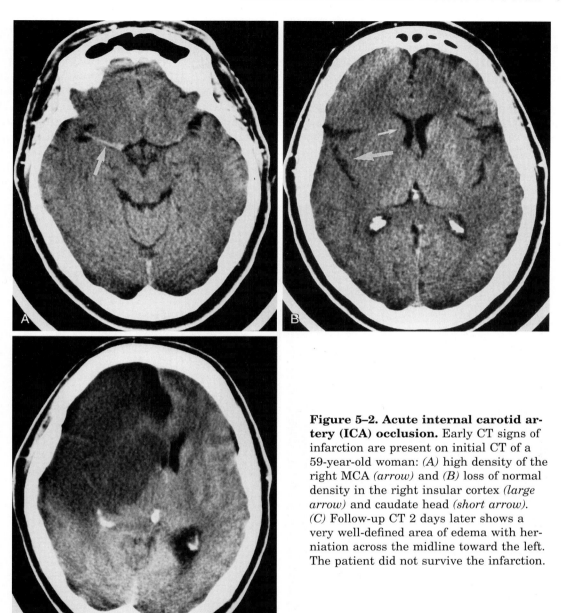

Figure 5–2. Acute internal carotid artery (ICA) occlusion. Early CT signs of infarction are present on initial CT of a 59-year-old woman: *(A)* high density of the right MCA *(arrow)* and *(B)* loss of normal density in the right insular cortex *(large arrow)* and caudate head *(short arrow)*. *(C)* Follow-up CT 2 days later shows a very well-defined area of edema with herniation across the midline toward the left. The patient did not survive the infarction.

vascular distribution, whereas embolic infarctions usually involve only a portion of a major arterial territory. However, the typical vascular distribution, often wedge-shaped and extending to the cortex, is a key element in the imaging diagnosis of either type of infarction.

MRI is more sensitive than CT for early changes of infarction. However, in the first few hours after vascular occlusion, MRI also may appear normal. Special techniques such as perfusion-weighted and diffusion-weighted imaging may provide earlier evidence of infarction. Although these techniques are now used primarily as research tools, their future clinical applications are promising.

Edema from ischemia or infarction, as from other causes, is seen on MRI as high signal intensity on T2-weighted images and low signal intensity on T1-weighted images. Mass effect is also apparent in the subacute stage. The identification of a vascular distribution is crucial in making the diagnosis (Figs. 5–3 to 5–5). MRI can be helpful when initial CT is insufficient or when the diagnosis remains in question.

Major Arterial Territories

The middle cerebral artery (MCA) and anterior cerebral artery (ACA) on each side arise from the terminal bifurcation of the respective internal carotid artery (ICA). The MCA is the most commonly affected large branch of the ICA in stroke. It supplies lateral portions of the frontal and parietal lobes and the superior portion of the temporal lobe

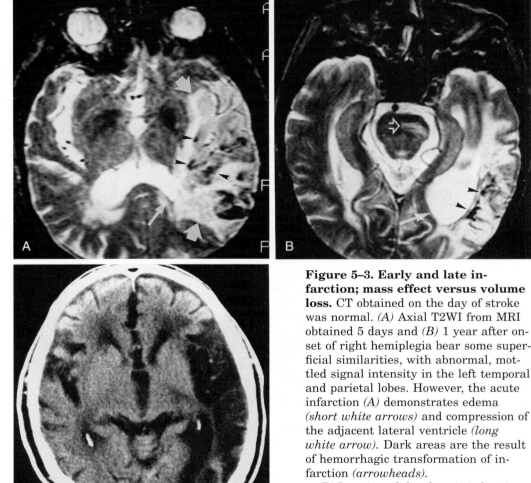

Figure 5–3. Early and late infarction; mass effect versus volume loss. CT obtained on the day of stroke was normal. *(A)* Axial T2WI from MRI obtained 5 days and *(B)* 1 year after onset of right hemiplegia bear some superficial similarities, with abnormal, mottled signal intensity in the left temporal and parietal lobes. However, the acute infarction *(A)* demonstrates edema *(short white arrows)* and compression of the adjacent lateral ventricle *(long white arrow).* Dark areas are the result of hemorrhagic transformation of infarction *(arrowheads).*

(B) Imaging of the chronic infarction shows encephalomalacia. Although high signal intensity is again present, it results from a different cause (gliosis) and, importantly, there is volume loss causing enlargement of the ventricle *(solid arrow).* Low signal intensity (dark) in the chronic infarction *(arrowheads)* is now the result of hemosiderin-laden macrophages in the areas of the old blood. Note also the high signal intensity in the left side of the pons *(open arrow)* from wallerian degeneration in the corticospinal tract. *(C)* The extent of encephalomalacia that resulted in wallerian degeneration is well demonstrated on a late CT scan.

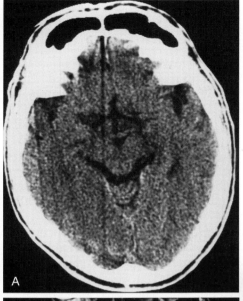

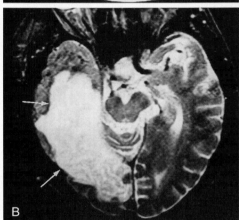

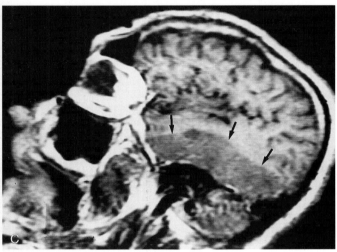

Figure 5–4. Acute posterior cerebral artery (PCA) infarction. *(A)* Initial CT shows only very subtle edema in the posterior right temporal and occipital lobes. *(B and C)* Distribution of abnormal signal intensity in the PCA territory is well demonstrated on MRI obtained 4 days later: high signal intensity on axial T2WI *(B, arrows)* and lower signal intensity than normal brain on sagittal T1WI, visible in the inferior temporal lobe *(C, arrows)*. The superior temporal lobe is supplied by the MCA, and the uncus is supplied by the anterior choroidal artery, and thus they are spared.

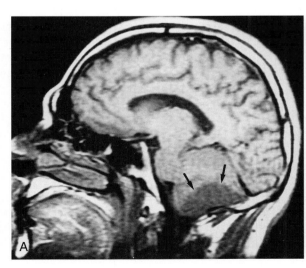

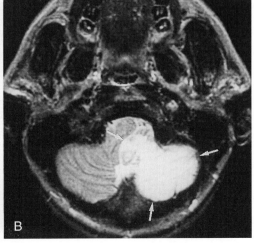

Figure 5–5. Acute posterior inferior cerebellar artery infarction. *(A and B)* MRI demonstrates edema in the left posterior inferior cerebellar artery territory in both sagittal T1WI *(A, arrows)* and axial T2WI *(B, arrows)*.

(see Fig. 5–3). The ACA supplies the medial aspect of the frontal lobe and extends posteriorly toward the parietal lobe. The posterior cerebral arteries (PCAs) are the terminal branches of the basilar artery and supply the occipital and inferior temporal lobes (see Fig. 5–4). Primary posterior supply from the anterior cerebral circulation (distal ICA) via a prominent posterior communicating artery (fetal origin of the PCA) is a common variant. The circle of Willis is highly variable in configuration and is complete in only 20 to 25 percent of cases. Collateral circulation has a great influence on the impact of arterial occlusion.

Cerebellar or brainstem infarction is also common. The three main arteries to the cerebellum (posterior inferior, anterior inferior, and superior cerebellar arteries) are somewhat variable in the size of the territory supplied by each, although the origin and general distribution are fairly consistent. The lateral medullary (Wallenberg) syndrome is caused by either posterior inferior cerebellar artery (PICA) or, more often, vertebral artery occlusion. Imaging results are similar to those found with supratentorial infarction, although the bone of the skull base can make CT in this region especially prone to artifact. MRI is thus superior to CT in diagnosis of infarction in the posterior fossa (see Fig. 5–5).

Infarctions involving small perforating arteries are also common. These include the lenticulostriate and thalamoperforating arteries, which supply the basal ganglia and thalami, and the small vessels to the brainstem. Lacunar infarctions involving the deep gray matter nuclei are often seen on CT and MRI as well-defined areas of abnormal fluid attenuation and signal intensity. Edema is present acutely, with progression ultimately to encephalomalacia, manifested on imaging studies by CSF attenuation or signal intensity.

Evolution of Infarction

As cell death and necrosis progress, edema and mass effect resolve. Volume loss (atrophy) then becomes apparent on imaging during the later stages of infarction (see Fig. 5–3). On CT this is seen as an area of low attenuation associated with enlarged sulci. Depending on the size, location, and age of the infarction, the nearby ventricular system may be enlarged (compensatory dilatation). With MRI, encephalomalacia is observed as volume loss and signal intensity similar to that of CSF on all pulse sequences. However, it is common to see adjacent areas, presumably representing gliosis, that demonstrate high signal intensity on both intermediate- and T2-weighted sequences.

Hemorrhagic transformation of an infarction can occur when a clot breaks down, resulting in reperfusion of damaged or dead brain tissue. On CT, acute hemorrhage has high attenuation. The MRI appearance of hemorrhage is more complex and is discussed in greater detail in Chapter 6. It is very common to see MRI evidence of hemorrhage in the cortical gyri in subacute or old infarction (see Fig. 5–3*B*). (Laminar necrosis, or partial cortical damage, without hemorrhage in an infarction can also produce high signal intensity on T1-weighted MR images.) Minor hemorrhage is of uncertain significance, although it must be considered in making decisions regarding anticoagulation. *The most important reason to look for hemorrhage in a patient who presents with a stroke is to detect other processes that can mimic the clinical presentation of infarction.* Such processes include hypertensive hemorrhage, arteriovenous malformation (AVM), and other causes of intracranial hemorrhage (Chapter 6). The clinical management of hemorrhagic stroke is quite different from that of bland infarction.

CAROTID ARTERY ATHEROSCLEROSIS

Previous infarction and transient ischemic attacks (TIAs) are among the indications for evaluation of the carotid arteries. The gold standard for carotid artery imaging is angiography, in which an iodinated contrast agent is injected through an arterial catheter (Fig. 5–6). Either digital subtraction an-

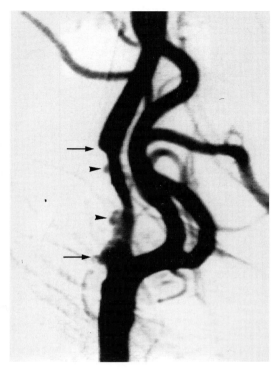

Figure 5–6. Carotid artery atherosclerosis.
A digital subtraction arteriogram was performed in a man who was having transient ischemic attacks. Lateral projection of the left common carotid bifurcation shows segmental stenosis of the proximal internal carotid artery *(between arrows)* because of a severely ulcerated plaque (arrowheads point to ulcerations).

giography (DSA) or cut-film technique can be used. In addition to excellent spatial detail, these techniques provide an opportunity to delineate the anatomy of the collateral circulation and the variations of intracerebral circulation. Various criteria for measurement of stenosis have been proposed.

Drawbacks of angiography include the risks of an adverse reaction to contrast agent, stroke, and complications of catheterization. Multiple views can be obtained but are limited to those projections used at the time of filming, usually two views, such as anteroposterior (AP) and lateral.

For screening purposes, noninvasive examinations are desirable. For proximal carotid atherosclerotic disease, ultrasound

examination or magnetic resonance angiography (MRA) are useful. Doppler ultrasound testing is widely available. This technique provides both anatomic information (narrowing of arteries) and functional information (velocities of blood within the arteries, waveforms, and comparison of systolic and diastolic velocities). MRA is a specific application of MRI that takes advantage of the fact that flowing blood is bright on gradient-recall images. Several techniques are available, but all rely on rendering blood vessels visible while suppressing background. Depending on the technique (two dimensional versus three dimensional, time-of-flight versus phase contrast), arterial or venous flow is selectively demonstrated by suppressing flow in one direction or by selecting a certain range of velocities to visualize. Usually no contrast agent is injected because the imaging technique is based on MRI properties of flowing blood (see Fig. 6–6B).

Choosing between Doppler ultrasound and MRA techniques for carotid evaluation depends on various factors, including availability and cost. Patient cooperation is more critical for MRA, which can be severely limited by patient motion. MRA is less dependent on operator skills than ultrasound examination. MRA alone is generally more expensive than ultrasound, but it is often obtained as an additional pulse sequence when a patient with symptoms of ischemia receives MRI of the brain. Although charges vary, the approximate cost difference is indicated by current Medicare reimbursement, which is approximately $230 for Doppler ultrasound examination of the carotid arteries and approximately $440 for cervical MRA. MRA can evaluate the vertebral arteries and intracranial circulation, which ultrasound testing cannot. Both techniques have some technical limitations. Although details are beyond the scope of this book, turbulent flow causes signal loss on MRI, which results in a tendency of MRA to overestimate stenosis. Advances in MRI technology may ameliorate this. Complete occlusions can make identification of remaining vessels with ultrasound examination difficult.

Dissecting aneurysm or dissection of

blood into the wall of an artery, which may also cause ischemia, is discussed in Chapter 6.

GLOBAL HYPOPERFUSION OR HYPOXIA

Temporary global ischemia of the brain results in a different pattern of damage. Border zone or watershed infarctions are located in the boundaries between major vascular territories. This occurs when diminished flow is sufficient to preserve the central region supplied by the vascular distribution but not the marginal areas. Typical patterns involve a strip between ACA and MCA in the frontal lobes and posteriorly between MCA and PCA territories (Fig.

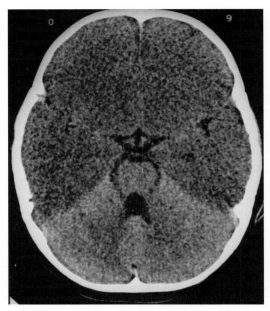

Figure 5–8. Global ischemia and CT reversal sign. CT scan of an infant who suffered cardiorespiratory arrest. There is diffuse low density of the cerebrum, compared with normal density of the cerebellum and brainstem.

5–7). Edema is present in this distribution acutely on CT or MRI. Because there is temporary reduction of flow rather than arterial occlusion, normal flow is re-established, and abnormal enhancement may occur early.

More prolonged periods of hypoperfusion or hypoxia, such as with cardiac or respiratory arrest, cause diffuse cerebral ischemia. The outcome is often poor. On CT, there is loss of gray-white differentiation, effacement of sulci, and lower density of the cerebrum compared with the cerebellum (CT reversal sign) (Fig. 5–8). MRI demonstrates diffuse cerebral edema (see Fig. 9–31B). Diffuse edema symmetrically involving the cortex can occasionally be difficult to appreciate. The basal ganglia are also often involved in diffuse hypoxic injury. More prominent involvement of the basal ganglia than the cortex is often observed in children and occasionally in adults (Fig. 5–9).

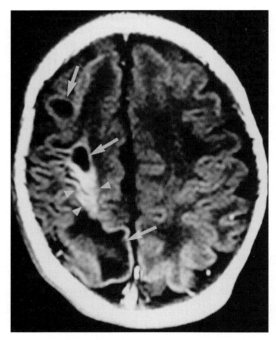

Figure 5–7. Border zone (watershed) infarction. MRI (axial T1WI) of a child who had a hypotensive event. Cystic changes *(arrows)* in a right cerebral hemisphere parasagittal distribution represent encephalomalacia in the border zone between anterior and middle cerebral artery territories. A small area of high signal intensity *(arrowheads)* is present from hemorrhage.

BRAIN DEATH

Prolonged periods of an inadequate supply of blood, glucose, or oxygen to the brain

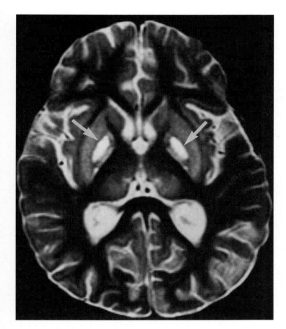

Figure 5–9. Global ischemia from near-drowning. MRI (axial T2WI) of a child who was resuscitated several minutes after falling into a pool. Markedly increased signal intensity within the globus pallidi *(arrows)* is from nearly complete necrosis, but high signal intensity from edema is also present within all of the other deep gray matter nuclei.

result in irreversible failure of cerebral function. Brain death is recognized both medically and legally as a condition that is equivalent to the death of the patient, even if the heart and other organs have not yet ceased activity. Criteria for determining brain death have been well described. They primarily involve clinical factors, such as the lack of any evidence of brainstem activity under defined conditions. Imaging is therefore supplemental, not primary, for brain death determination. On angiography, there is no intracranial blood flow when intracranial pressure exceeds or equals arterial pressure.

Nuclear medicine studies are also helpful in confirming brain death (Fig. 5–10). When there is no detectable intracranial blood flow with venous injection of a radionuclide, all of the common carotid blood flow is diverted to the extracranial tissues. Increased extracranial flow (and the absence of intra-

cranial flow) causes a "hot nose" sign, with considerable radionuclide activity identified in the nose and face.

MRI has been described more recently as another modality that can confirm the absence of intracranial blood flow. Usually only one imaging study is necessary, and the purpose is to confirm the clinical results.

VENOUS INFARCTION

Venous infarction is uncommon but important. It usually results from dural sinus thrombosis, but deep cerebral venous thrombosis can also occur. In infants, dehydration is the most common predisposing factor. In adults, altered coagulation states, such as that from oral contraceptive use, are risk factors for venous sinus thrombosis. Infection near a dural sinus, especially otitis or mastoiditis, can cause a septic thrombophlebitis. Skull fracture involving a dural sinus can also cause thrombosis. Clinical manifestations can be insidious and subtle. A small or nonoccluding area of dural sinus thrombosis, or one transverse sinus thrombosed with the other side remaining open, can be asymptomatic. However, with involvement of enough of the venous drainage system to cause venous congestion, ischemia and infarction can ensue. Patchy areas of edema are often present in the white matter on CT or MRI, usually bilaterally, and multifocal hemorrhage may also occur (Fig. 5–11). The distribution does not correspond to an arterial territory, and thus it is important to remember the possibility of venous infarction when an unusual distribution of ischemia is present.

To diagnose sinus thrombosis, angiography is definitive, with the involved portion of the dural sinuses not visualized in the venous phase (see Fig. 5–11A). Less invasive tests are often diagnostic. A classic appearance of superior sagittal thrombosis on contrast-enhanced CT is the empty delta sign, with dense contrast surrounding and outlining the less dense thrombus in the middle. MRI has the advantage of multiple planes and sensitivity to both flowing blood and various stages of thrombus. Blood flow

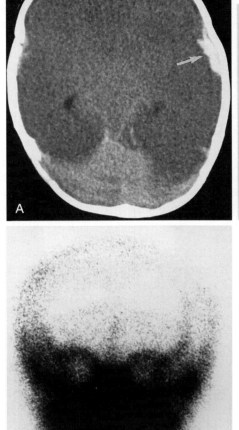

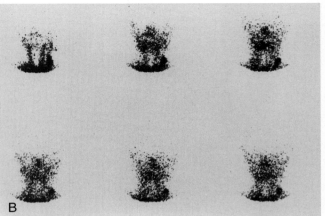

Figure 5–10. Brain death. *(A)* CT scan of a victim of child abuse shows diffuse low density of the cerebrum, denser cerebellum, and subdural blood *(arrow)* overlying the left hemisphere. *(B and C)* Radionuclide scan of the brain with technetium-99m was performed. Dynamic *(B)* and static images *(C)* show immediate flow through the common and external carotid arteries to the face, but no appreciable intracranial flow.

within the dural sinuses can normally be slow, with resultant variable appearance on MRI. However, careful inspection of the sinuses in multiple planes and using different pulse sequences usually permits identification of a thrombosed dural sinus. After several days, when methemoglobin is present, the appearance is characteristic (Fig. 5–12). MRA using inferior saturation bands to negate arterial signal (for time-of-flight technique) or slow-flow technique (for phase contrast studies) can also help, and intravenous contrast material administration is occasionally beneficial.

METABOLIC CONDITIONS RESULTING IN FOCAL BRAIN DAMAGE

Several toxins, especially carbon monoxide, cyanide, methanol, and ethylene glycol, result in inadequate tissue oxygenation. The basal ganglia are often particularly susceptible to damage after poisoning with these agents. CT and MRI both demonstrate findings of symmetric edema in the basal ganglia, with MRI being more sensitive. If cell death occurs, encephalomalacia follows.

Osmotic myelinolysis is an uncommon

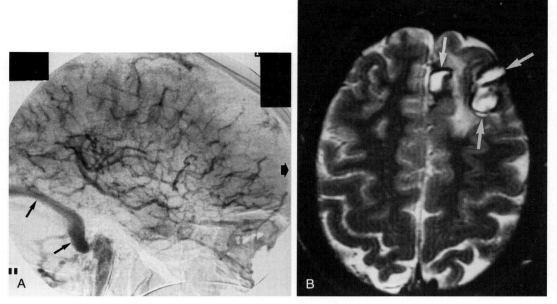

Figure 5–11. Venous infarction from superior sagittal thrombosis. *(A)* Venous phase of angiogram, in a lateral projection from internal carotid injection, shows only a small amount of contrast medium within the superior sagittal sinus, which is almost entirely thrombosed. Transverse and sigmoid sinuses *(arrows)* and internal jugular vein are present. (Large arrow points anterior.) *(B)* Later MRI (T2WI) shows subacute hemorrhage *(arrows)* in the left frontal lobe, as well as abnormal signal intensity in the adjacent white matter.

condition that results in a striking imaging appearance. The mechanism of injury is not ischemia but loss of myelin, usually occurring several days after metabolic disturbances. Rapid correction of hyponatremia is a particularly common clinical setting. Classically, the patient begins to recover from neurologic symptoms related to severe hyponatremia, then the condition worsens after several days and the patient may enter a locked-in state. The central pons is the most common location, hence the term *central pontine myelinolysis*. The broader term *osmotic myelinolysis* has been recom-

Figure 5–12. Cerebral venous thrombosis. Sagittal MRI (noncontrast T1WI) of an infant who had deep cerebral venous thrombosis. Methemoglobin signal (high signal intensity) is visible in a thrombosed internal cerebral vein *(arrow)*.

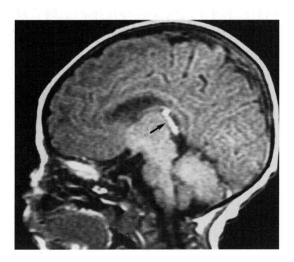

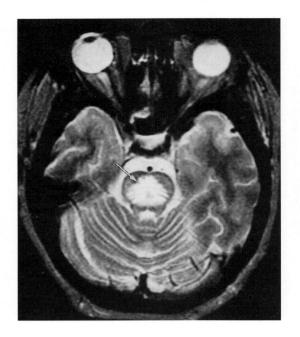

Figure 5–13. Osmotic (central pontine) myelinolysis. Axial T2WI from MRI of a 30-year-old alcoholic whose condition deteriorated to a locked-in state several days after admission. The patient initially was severely hyponatremic. Prominent high signal intensity is present within the pons *(arrow),* with a rim of surrounding tissue spared. Note also the alcohol-related cerebellar atrophy, with prominent folia.

mended, because extrapontine involvement, especially in the basal ganglia, can also occur. MRI is the most sensitive imaging test (Fig. 5–13). High signal intensity on T2-weighted images and low signal on T1-weighted images are seen in the central pons and occasionally elsewhere. The corticospinal tracts can be spared.

6

Intracranial Hemorrhage and Related Vascular Diseases

Nonocclusive vascular diseases of the brain are discussed in this chapter. Many of these are associated with intracranial hemorrhage. Common causes of intracranial hemorrhage are listed in Table 6–1. CT is usually the first imaging test obtained when acute intracranial hemorrhage is suspected. MRI is often more helpful during later stages or during follow-up of hemorrhage. Magnetic resonance angiography (MRA) is becoming increasingly useful for visualizing blood vessels. For this group of vascular diseases in particular, however, conventional (intra-arterial, catheter-based) angiography may be necessary for diagnosis and characterization of the underlying pathologic process. Particularly for arteriovenous malformations (AVMs), endovascular therapy (catheter-delivered intervention) is often part of a team approach to treatment.

INTRACRANIAL HEMORRHAGE

Intracranial hemorrhage should be described in terms of both location and appearance. Extra-axial hemorrhage can be epidural, subdural, or subarachnoid in location. Epidural and subdural hematomas are usually the result of trauma; appearance and examples have been presented in Chapter 2. Subdural hematomas in the elderly

can result from unrecognized, sometimes trivial, trauma. In children, any type of intracranial hemorrhage without adequate explanation should bring to mind the possibility of child abuse (nonaccidental trauma).

Subarachnoid Hemorrhage

The most common causes of subarachnoid hemorrhage (SAH) are trauma (Chapter 2) and ruptured cerebral aneurysm. It is extremely important to recognize SAH, because it may be the only CT sign of a ruptured aneurysm. CT shows increased attenuation within the sulci or cisterns (Fig. 6–1). Subtly increased density or very symmetric patterns of SAH may be difficult to appreciate on CT. The distribution of the blood often provides a clue to the source of the hemorrhage.

SAH can occasionally be observed on T1-weighted MRI. In general, however, SAH is difficult to identify by MRI and remains an area of relative weakness for MRI as compared with CT.

Communicating hydrocephalus is a complication commonly resulting from diffuse SAH and may require surgical intervention. It may occur soon after SAH or as a late complication.

Intraventricular Hemorrhage

Intraventricular hemorrhage (IVH) is associated with multiple etiologies. These in-

TABLE 6–1. **Causes of Intracranial Hemorrhage**

Trauma
    Clear history of trauma
    Nonaccidental trauma (child abuse, spouse
      abuse)
Aneurysm
    "Berry"
    Mycotic
    Traumatic
Vascular malformations
    AVM
    Cavernous angioma
    Dural AVF
    (Venous angioma [usually does not bleed])
    (Capillary telangiectasia [rarely bleeds])
    Vein of Galen malformation
Hypertension
Amyloid angiopathy
Neoplasm
    Metastatic
      Especially renal, melanoma, choriocarcinoma,
        lung
    Primary brain (glioblastoma multiforme)
    Pituitary adenoma
Prematurity, germinal matrix hemorrhage
Infarction with hemorrhagic transformation
Venous infarction
Infection
    Herpes (the presence of intracranial hemorrhage
      is not a sensitive indicator for herpes but is
      strongly suggestive of herpes when it does
      occur in the setting of infection)
Coagulopathy
Drugs (cocaine, etc.)

clude trauma, systemic hypertension, ruptured aneurysm, and AVM. Acute IVH is recognized on CT as an area of much higher attenuation (whiter) than that of cerebrospinal fluid (CSF). The choroid plexus is very frequently calcified and must be differentiated on CT from intraventricular blood. Typical location and symmetry are helpful signs in recognizing calcified choroid plexus. A clot within the ventricular system may be somewhat irregular in shape, often filling or partially filling a ventricle (Fig. 6–2). Blood commonly assumes a dependent position within the ventricle, creating a CSF-blood layer. The occipital horns of the lateral ventricles are the most common locations for this phenomenon. It is common for blood to extend through the ventricular system and into the subarachnoid space. Intraventricular blood is usually quite different in signal intensity from CSF on MRI. Hydrocephalus is a possible complication of IVH.

Parenchymal Hemorrhage

Causes of parenchymal hemorrhage include those listed for IVH, as well as hemorrhage into a neoplasm and hemorrhagic infarction. When hemorrhage is present within the brain itself, the location (hemisphere, basal ganglia, cerebellum, brainstem) is important. Specific locations are common with certain pathologic processes, such as hypertensive hemorrhage in the basal ganglia and cerebellum, and lobar hemorrhage with amyloid angiopathy. The extent of mass effect should also be noted, including factors such as amount of surrounding edema, effect on the ventricular system, and shift of the midline (see Fig. 6–2).

CT APPEARANCE OF HEMORRHAGE

Intracranial blood usually passes through a simple progression on CT. Initially it has higher attenuation than the brain but less than bone, with Hounsfield or attenuation units of approximately 35 to 80 (Figs. 6–1*A*, 6–2, 6–3). The high attenuation of blood is primarily the result of protein; iron alone is not responsible for the CT appearance. Over several days to weeks, there is a gradual decrease in attenuation. For this reason, subacute hemorrhage can be especially difficult to recognize on CT. For example, subdural hematomas may be nearly isodense compared with brain at 1 to 2 weeks (see Fig. 2–5), and signs other than attenuation alone (e.g., mass effect) must be sought (see Fig. 2–4). With additional time there is a further decrease in attenuation, becoming lower than that of brain. Blood in normal CSF-containing spaces (intraventricular and subarachnoid hemorrhage) is usually resorbed before passing through these stages, although actual clot takes longer to evolve. Ultimately, intraparenchymal blood

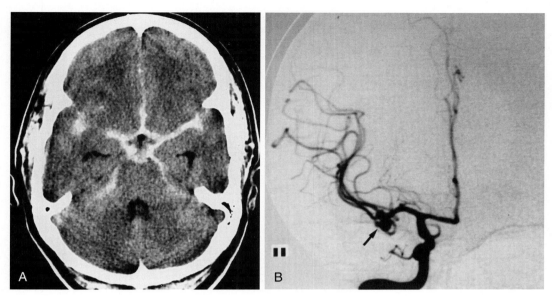

Figure 6–1. Subarachnoid hemorrhage and berry aneurysm. *(A)* Nonenhanced CT of a 43-year-old hypertensive woman who experienced sudden onset of severe headache shows high-attenuation subarachnoid hemorrhage in the cisterns around the base of brain. *(B)* Angiography was performed; anteroposterior view of a right internal carotid injection shows a multilobulated aneurysm *(arrow)* at the bifurcation of the middle cerebral artery.

Figure 6–2. Intracranial hemorrhage from hypertension. Nonenhanced CT shows large hemorrhage in the right thalamus that has extended into the ventricular system. A blood-CSF level is present in the lateral ventricle. (From Mettler F: Essentials of Radiology. Philadelphia, WB Saunders, 1995, p 24.)

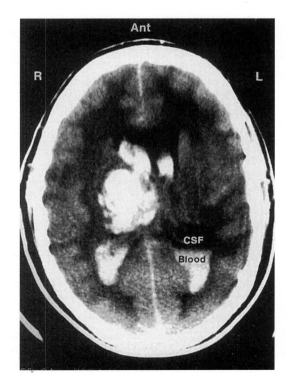

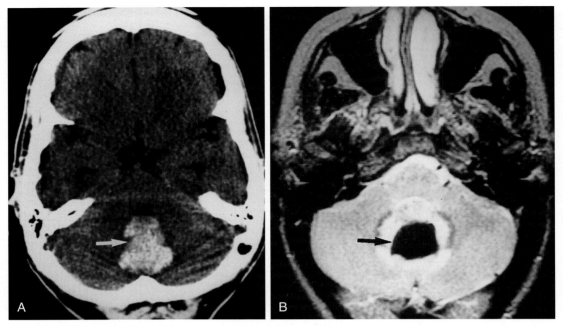

Figure 6–3. Acute hemorrhage on CT and MRI. *(A)* On nonenhanced CT, acute cerebellar hemorrhage appears bright *(arrow)*. *(B)* On MRI (axial T2WI) obtained the next day, acute blood is seen as a region of very low signal intensity *(arrow)*.

is resorbed but may leave encephalomalacia (loss of brain tissue, manifested on CT by low attenuation) or calcification (high attenuation on CT).

MRI APPEARANCE OF HEMORRHAGE

The appearance of blood on MRI is much more complex, and extensive reviews of this subject are available. Many factors affect this appearance, including the changes in hemoglobin and the attendant paramagnetic state of iron atoms, clot shrinkage with loss of water, rupture of red cell membranes, and field strength of the imaging system. A simplified summary follows (Table 6–2).

The MRI appearance of very acute bleeding within the first few hours, has been described variably, perhaps depending on field strength of the MRI system. One reason for the poor characterization is that for many years acutely ill patients were seldom scanned with MRI within minutes to hours of hemorrhage onset. High signal intensity is usually present on T2-weighted images and occasionally on T1-weighted images.

Acute Hemorrhage

Acute hemorrhage, that is, within a few hours to days of bleeding, is typically of very low signal intensity on T2-weighted images and mildly decreased intensity on T1-weighted images (see Fig. 6–3B). In part this results from predominance of deoxyhemoglobin, which has four unpaired electrons but is shielded by the protein configuration of globin from T1-shortening effects. Edema, manifested as high signal intensity on T2-weighted images, is observed around the hematoma soon after hemorrhage.

Subacute Hemorrhage

Further evolution of MRI changes begins at the periphery of a hematoma. As deoxyhemoglobin changes to methemoglobin, high signal intensity appears on the T1-weighted images. Because of its paramagnetic nature (five unpaired electrons), methemoglobin

TABLE 6–2. **Appearance of Blood on MRI***

Acute	T1:	Isointense to mildly hypointense
(Deoxyhemoglobin)	T2:	Very hypointense
Early subacute	T1:	Increasing hyperintensity
(Intracellular methemoglobin)	T2:	Hypointense initially, changing to isointense
Late subacute	T1:	Hyperintense
(Extracellular methemoglobin)	T2:	Hyperintense centrally
		A thin, hypointense rim appears
Chronic	T1:	Hyperintensity decreases over time
(Hemosiderin-laden	T2:	Rim of hypointensity increases, central hyperintensity
macrophages remain)		decreases, leaving only a low signal intensity scar

*General guide only; the appearance of blood on MRI is very complex (see text).

causes marked T1 shortening, resulting in high signal intensity on both T1- and T2-weighted (short- and long-echo) sequences. However, local field inhomogeneity caused by hemoglobin within intact red blood cells results in very rapid loss of phase coherence, that is, a very short T2 and low signal intensity on T2-weighted images. Early subacute hematoma, still with intact red blood cells (intracellular methemoglobin), thus

has a striking appearance: very bright on T1-weighted images and very dark on T2-weighted images (Fig. 6–4).

As red cell membranes break down, there is less impact on the spin-spin (T2) interactions, and the T1-shortening effect predominates even on long TR/long TE images. Late subacute to chronic hematomas (extracellular methemoglobin) have one of the easiest appearances to recognize on MRI, with very

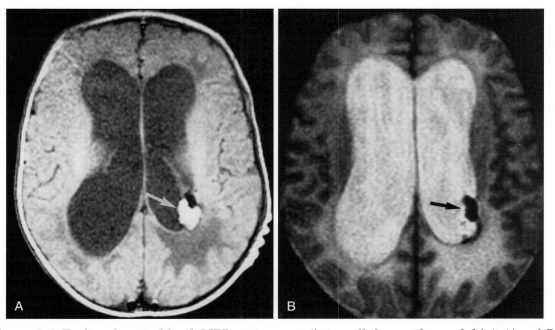

Figure 6–4. Early subacute blood, MRI appearance (intracellular methemoglobin). (*A* and *B*) MRI of an infant who had an intraventricular hemorrhage and subsequent hydrocephalus shows a clot within the left lateral ventricle *(arrows)*. Most of the clot has high signal intensity on the T1WI *(A)* and very low signal intensity on the T2WI *(B)*, which is consistent with intracellular methemoglobin.

high signal intensity on all spin-echo sequences (Fig. 6–5).

Chronic Hemorrhage

The normal response to parenchymal hemorrhage results in further degradation of methemoglobin. Hemosiderin-laden macrophages result in a dark ring around a hematoma on T2-weighted images, while there is further loss of the bright methemoglobin. Eventually only a small scar of low signal intensity hemosiderin may remain (see Figs. 5–3*B*, 6–11).

Other Factors

As mentioned above, the presented scheme is simplified. Various factors, in addition to oxygenation state of hemoglobin, also come into play. Moreover, the cause of the hemorrhage can affect the MRI appearance. Hemorrhagic neoplasms, for example, may have a complex appearance (see Fig. 6–15), and hemorrhage within a poorly vascularized tumor may evolve more slowly than might be expected. AVMs and, especially, cavernous angiomas often are associated with episodes of repeated bleeding, causing a complex appearance. Associated abnormal blood vessels, such as from an AVM, further complicate imaging. Depending on the flow velocity, blood within vessels may demonstrate no signal (high flow) or variable signal (low flow). Band-like artifacts in the phase-encoding direction can result from flow (see Fig. 4–22). Flowing blood usually

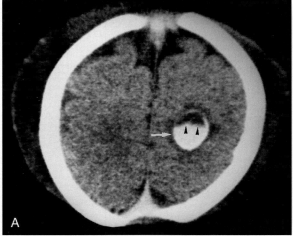
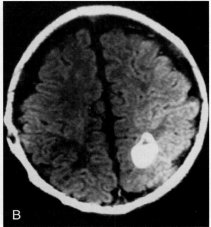
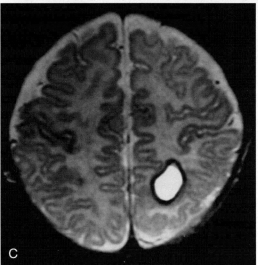

Figure 6–5. Subacute hemorrhage on MRI. *(A)* Nonenhanced CT scan of an infant shows acute (dense) hemorrhage in the left cerebral hemisphere *(arrow)*. A hematocrit effect is seen, with a dependent layer *(arrowheads)*. *(B* and *C)* MRI was obtained 3 weeks later. Subacute hemorrhage is seen as bright on both axial T1WI *(B)* and axial T2WI *(C)*. A thin rim of low signal intensity (hemosiderin) is beginning to appear around the hematoma on the T2WI *(C)*.

results in high signal intensity on gradient-recall type pulse sequences.

Despite the apparent complexity of the MRI appearance of hemorrhage, the usual sequence of changes of hemorrhage on MRI is fairly consistent (Table 6–2). Details such as those described earlier can add further helpful information. MRI is thus very useful for the detection and characterization of intracranial hemorrhage.

Subacute hematomas often demonstrate peripheral contrast enhancement on either CT or MRI and must be included in the differential diagnosis of ring-enhancing masses (see Table 4–1).

CT and MRI are complementary regarding the evaluation of hemorrhage, and follow-up scans can be particularly helpful for the evaluation of the typical changes of evolving hemorrhage.

INTRACRANIAL ANEURYSM

Saccular aneurysms, often termed *berry aneurysms,* are outpouchings of the wall of an artery that occur at a bifurcation. They are not congenital, as was once thought, but are probably related to hemodynamic stresses at arterial bifurcations and to vascular degeneration. All walls of the artery are involved, although tunica media is usually absent within the aneurysm itself. The incidence of intracranial aneurysms in the general adult population is difficult to determine with certainty. Studies based on autopsy series and angiographic results report a 3 to 5 percent incidence. In addition to the spontaneous incidence, there is an increased association of intracranial aneurysms with several conditions, including polycystic kidney disease, aortic coarctation, and connective tissue diseases such as Marfan disease.

Presentation of Intracranial Aneurysm

The greatest risk of berry aneurysm is rupture. The consequences are often catastrophic. Subarachnoid hemorrhage nearly always occurs, accompanied by severe headache and often loss of consciousness. Spasm of other cerebral arteries is common, and the ischemia or infarction that follows is a major cause of morbidity and mortality. Intraparenchymal and intraventricular hemorrhage are not uncommon. The intraparenchymal hemorrhage causes focal central nervous system deficits and mass effect, and both intraventricular and subarachnoid hemorrhage can lead to hydrocephalus. For patients who survive the initial hemorrhage, there is a high rate of rebleeding if the aneurysm is not treated (up to 50% in the first 6 months). Rebleeding occurs most frequently in the first few days following the initial hemorrhage. Despite advances in therapy, the mortality rate remains approximately 50 percent.

Other presentations of intracranial aneurysms are less common. An aneurysm can cause cranial nerve abnormalities by compression of the cisternal segment of the nerve. For example, an aneurysm of the posterior communicating artery often causes third cranial nerve palsy. Cavernous sinus aneurysms often cause neuropathies of the adjacent cranial nerves (three through six) (see Fig. 4–22). Aneurysms larger than 2.5 cm in diameter are referred to as *giant aneurysms,* and patients often present because of mass effect rather than hemorrhage. Symptoms such as those described earlier, in addition to the associated discomfort, are important clues to the possible presence of a life-threatening aneurysm.

Imaging the Patient with Acute Rupture of an Aneurysm

The approach to imaging depends to some extent on the presentation, particularly whether or not an aneurysm has ruptured. The Hunt and Hess grading system of SAH is a widely used means of reporting the patient's neurologic status (Table 6–3). Nonenhanced CT is usually the most appropriate first imaging test obtained on such patients, who are often comatose or severely impaired (Fig. 6–1A). The goal is to detect SAH as well as to evaluate for parenchymal damage and hydrocephalus. CT is very sensitive to SAH *but not 100 percent* sensitive. Lumbar puncture can reveal SAH in those

TABLE 6–3. **Hunt-Hess Clinical Grading System for Subarachnoid Hemorrhage**

Grade 1	Asymptomatic or mild headache
Grade 2	Moderate to severe headache, cranial nerve (oculomotor) palsy, or nuchal rigidity
Grade 3	Lethargy, confusion, or mild focal deficit
Grade 4	Stupor, moderate to severe hemiparesis, or early decerebrate rigidity
Grade 5	Coma or moribund appearance or decerebrate rigidity

cases when the cranial CT scan is normal (up to 10%).

SAH on CT is manifested as high attenuation within the sulci or cisterns, instead of low-density CSF. The distribution can sometimes provide information about the location of an aneurysm. For example, anterior communicating artery aneurysms lead to bleeding within the nearby cistern of the lamina terminalis and a predominant frontal pattern of blood. Middle cerebral artery aneurysms often cause prominent sylvian fissure SAH. However, SAH often spreads readily, limiting the value of this localizing information.

Other important observations that may be noted on CT following rupture of an aneurysm include blood in the ventricles or parenchyma and hydrocephalus. Acute intraventricular and parenchymal blood also demonstrates high attenuation, appearing bright on CT. Hydrocephalus commonly contributes to the neurologic morbidity of these patients.

When clinical presentation and CT findings indicate a probable ruptured aneurysm, angiography is usually the next imaging test undertaken. Urgency depends on planned surgical intervention. Because of the potential for arterial vasospasm or rebleeding, surgery to clip an aneurysm is usually performed either immediately (in which case angiography is indicated emergently) or up to 1 to 3 weeks later. The risk of vasospasm is greatest from 3 days to 2 weeks following rupture. With angiography, the carotid and vertebral arteries are catheterized and images are obtained during injection of iodinated contrast material. More than one projection must be obtained, and occasionally several are necessary. Either cut-film or digital subtraction angiography (DSA) technique is satisfactory with good equipment, the latter having the advantages of shorter processing times and lower contrast loads.

Angiographic Findings

A saccular aneurysm appears on angiography as a rounded structure at an arterial bifurcation (see Fig. 6–1*B*). A more complex or lobulated appearance may occasionally be present. The majority arise from the circle of Willis or middle cerebral artery bifurcation. The anterior communicating artery, posterior communicating artery origin, and middle cerebral artery bifurcation are especially common locations. Posterior circulation aneurysms, such as those arising from the basilar artery tip and the posterior inferior cerebellar artery bifurcation from the vertebral artery, account for a smaller proportion (about 10%) of aneurysms. Because greater than 15 percent of aneurysm patients have more than one aneurysm, it is important not to assume that the responsible lesion has been found once one aneurysm has been identified. Generally, all major intracranial arteries should be evaluated. If more than one aneurysm is found, several clues can suggest which one was most likely to have bled. These include larger size, lobulated contour, location of SAH or surrounding clot on CT, proximity of vasospasm, and, rarely, direct visualization of extravasation. Because of arterial spasm and technical limitations, a small number of cases may have negative results on initial angiography. Repeat angiography in 1 to 3 weeks after hemorrhage is indicated if SAH is definite by CT or lumbar puncture.

Imaging the Patient with an Unruptured Aneurysm

The patient with an incidentally discovered or suspected aneurysm presents different challenges. An unruptured intracranial aneurysm has approximately a 2 percent risk of rupture per year. Because this risk rate is cumulative, surgery is likely to be a favorable choice for an otherwise healthy patient. Aneurysms can occasionally be detected on CT or MRI. CT is usually not used for this purpose because other techniques are more sensitive. However, the following observations on CT performed for other purposes should prompt further evaluation for aneurysm. An aneurysm appears on CT as a round, oval, or lobulated area similar in attenuation to blood vessels but larger than the adjacent arteries, and occurs in an appropriate location such as near the circle of Willis (Fig. 6–6*A*). Calcification is occasionally present within an aneurysm.

As previously mentioned, flowing blood has complex characteristics on MRI. On spin-echo MRI sequences, an aneurysm also has a round contour and lies near arterial bifurcations. However, the signal intensity can vary, with signal void in areas of rapid flow, variable signal in areas of slower or turbulent flow, and signal characteristics of old hematoma in clot that may be present within the residual lumen of the aneurysm. There is often an associated band of artifact in the phase-encoding direction caused by turbulent flow within the aneurysm (see Fig. 4–22).

High signal intensity results from flowing blood on gradient-recall pulse sequences. This is the basis for MRA techniques. Methods for MRA are continuing to improve, and high-quality MRA may be an appropriate screening examination for some patients suspected of having an aneurysm (Fig. 6–6*B*). CT angiography is an emerging and promising technique that may prove to be useful in some situations. However, catheter-based arterial angiography remains the standard for imaging when there is strong suspicion of aneurysm. Because there is a small risk of major complications from angiography, the level of suspicion of aneurysm must be carefully evaluated. Nevertheless, complications of angiography are far less than those of aneurysm rupture.

Other Aneurysms

Other types of aneurysms can also occur, although less frequently. Mycotic aneurysms result from infection within and weakening of the arterial wall. They are often more peripheral in location than saccular aneurysms and may be multiple. Pen-

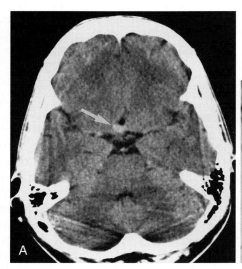
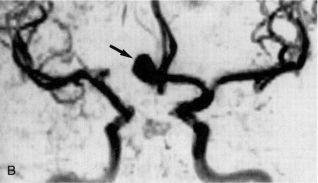

Figure 6–6. Incidental detection of aneurysm. (*A*) Nonenhanced CT obtained in a 40-year-old woman revealed an oval area of higher attenuation than brain in the expected region of the anterior communicating artery *(arrow)*. (*B*) MRA, on AP projection, confirms the presence of an aneurysm *(arrow)*. (The proximal segment of the right anterior cerebral artery is missing or atretic, which is a variant of the circle of Willis.)

etrating trauma can lead to pseudoaneurysm formation if an arterial wall is damaged but surrounding clot contains the blood flow and prevents extravasation. Closed head injuries (without penetrating injury) can also lead to torn vessel walls and pseudoaneurysm formation, especially at locations where arteries lie adjacent to rigid structures, such as the falx cerebri. These aneurysms also have serious clinical implications. Angiography is the most sensitive imaging test for these lesions. Severe atherosclerosis can lead to fusiform aneurysm formation in ectatic (enlarged, tortuous) arteries. This is especially common in the vertebrobasilar system (dolichoectastia) in elderly patients. Mass effect, as well as hemorrhage, are common complications. Treatment can be quite difficult because penetrating branches to the brainstem often exist and, unlike saccular aneurysms, there is no neck or narrow base that can be clipped.

DISSECTING ANEURYSMS

Injury to the intima of an artery can lead to bleeding into the vessel wall itself and can cause a dissecting aneurysm or dissection without aneurysm formation. Extracranial portions of the carotid and vertebral arteries are more often involved than intracranial segments. Penetrating trauma and abrupt stretching of the artery, as with motor vehicle accident deceleration injuries or neck manipulation, may cause dissection. Vasculitis and other vasculopathies such as fibromuscular dysplasia can be associated with dissection. Some cases are apparently spontaneous in that a precipitating factor is not identified. The remaining true lumen of the artery is often narrowed, and ischemic symptoms are common.

Angiography or MRA can be used to evaluate a suspected dissecting aneurysm. Appearance on angiography includes tapered vessel narrowing, a flap within the lumen, and visualization of an entry site into the false channel (Fig. 6–7). Similar findings can be sought on MRA. The presence of a peripheral crescent of hematoma around a

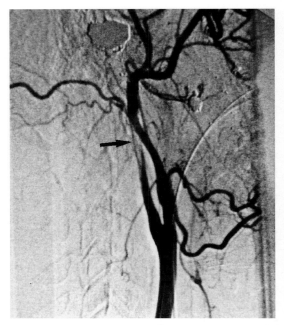

Figure 6–7. Traumatic carotid artery dissection. Arteriogram of a 17-year-old youth who was shot in the face. Lateral projection from a digital subtraction arteriogram shows narrowing of the cervical portion of the internal carotid artery *(arrow)*. Subtraction artifact from some bullet fragments is visible near the top of the image.

narrowed arterial lumen on axial MRI is especially helpful. The source images from which MRA images are reconstructed should always be inspected for this occurrence.

VASCULAR MALFORMATIONS

Vascular malformations are classified into four pathologic types: arteriovenous malformations (AVMs), cavernous angiomas, venous angiomas, and capillary telangiectasias. AVMs are further classified according to the vascular supply as pial, dural, or mixed. The risk of hemorrhage and other complications differs considerably for these different malformations.

Arteriovenous Malformations

Pial AVMs are caused by an abnormal connection between arteries and veins in the brain. A tangle of vessels is typically present. Multiple feeding arteries are not uncommon. The high flow into veins causes enlargement and alteration in the walls. Because of the abnormal flow patterns, aneurysmal components are often present within the AVM. Hemorrhage is a major risk, but the high flow shunted through the AVM can also cause ischemia to the nearby brain that is deprived of normal blood flow. As a result, gliosis may be present in adjacent brain tissue. Size, location, and venous drainage pattern of an AVM are all important factors in predicting the natural history and risks of an AVM. A widely used grading scheme for AVMs is presented in Table 6–4. The risk accompanying surgery is related to the grade of the AVM.

Imaging Appearance of AVM

Pial malformations can be suggested by CT or MRI, but angiography is often necessary to diagnose and characterize them. The hallmark is a tangle of vessels (Fig. 6–8). Multiple vessels with attenuation characteristics of arteries and veins are identified

TABLE 6–4. **Spetzler Grading System* for Arteriovenous Malformations (AVMs)**

Characteristics	Points
Size	
<3 cm	1
3–6 cm	2
>6 cm	3
Eloquence of adjacent brain	
Noneloquent	0
Eloquent	1
(Includes sensorimotor, language, or visual cortex; hypothalamus, thalamus; internal capsule; brainstem; cerebral peduncles; deep cerebellar nuclei)	
Venous drainage pattern	
Superficial only	0
Deep drainage	1

*Grade is the sum of the score for the three features above (size, eloquence of adjacent brain, and venous drainage pattern), from 1 to 5.
A score of 6 has been used for very large (e.g., hemispheric) AVMs.

on CT. A similar appearance is observed on MRI, but the signal intensity varies depending on the direction and velocity of blood flow (Fig. 6–9). Rapidly flowing blood is associated with no signal on spin-echo techniques, but some parts of an AVM can have slowly flowing blood, which yields variable signal intensity. Phase-encoding pulsation artifacts may be present, which are seen as a band-like, indistinct region in the phase-encoding direction. Gradient echo techniques can help by highlighting blood vessels. MRA provides another method of depicting an AVM.

Angiography is definitive and yields additional information. Direct arterial-to-venous connections are visible, with rapid filling of the venous system. Associated aneurysms are more readily identified. Subselective catheterization of the different arteries supplying an AVM, with magnification views, can be very helpful in planning therapy.

Treatment of AVMs is not discussed here in detail. Briefly, three techniques are available, and a combination of these is often employed. Surgery is often necessary to eliminate the risks of an AVM but can be very difficult in deep locations. Endovascular therapy involves deposition of glue or embolic material within the nidus of an AVM from an arterial catheter. It is often performed as part of a combined or staged surgical approach. Focused radiation therapy is also effective in some cases, especially if the AVM is not too large.

Dural arteriovenous fistulae arise within the walls of dural sinuses. There is direct shunting of blood from the arterial to venous systems. Previous dural sinus thrombosis may be an underlying factor in some cases. The dural sinuses around the skull base are most often involved, especially the transverse, sigmoid, and cavernous sinuses. The arteries supplying these dural lesions are most often external carotid branches, and tentorial and posterior meningeal branches from the internal carotid and vertebral arteries, respectively. Symptoms include bruits and cranial nerve deficits. Intracranial hemorrhage is not common but is more likely if venous varices are present or if cortical venous occlusion leads to venous infarction. Angiography is the best imaging

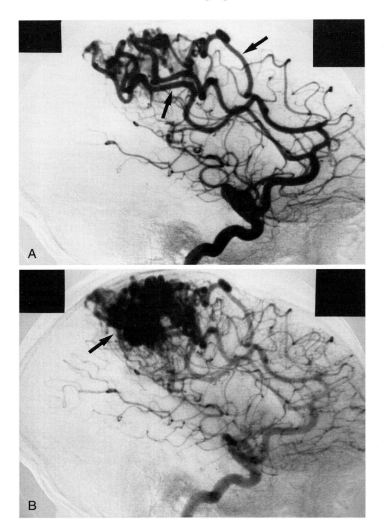

Figure 6–8. Pial arteriovenous malformation. A large left cerebral hemisphere AVM has arterial supply from several large branches. *(A)* Lateral projection from arteriogram, mid-arterial phase, shows enlarged MCA branches *(arrows)*. *(B)* A later image shows a dense tangle of vessels *(arrow)*.

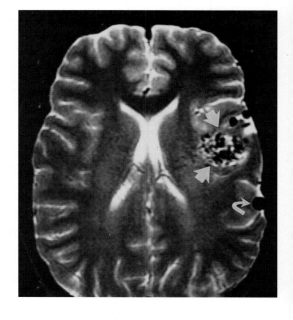

Figure 6–9. Arteriovenous malformation (AVM). MRI (axial T2WI) shows multiple areas of signal void within a left frontal lobe AVM *(straight arrows)*. A large, draining cortical vein is visible on the surface of the brain *(curved arrow)*.

test for displaying details of the malformation and for planning therapy (Fig. 6–10).

Cavernous Angioma

Cavernous angiomas are formed of sinusoidal blood vessels without normal intervening brain tissue. Blood flow is very slow, which means that they are nearly always angiographically occult. There is a tendency for repeated hemorrhage within the malformation. Hemorrhage is responsible for the typical imaging features, especially on MRI. A subcortical location is most common, but angiomas can occur anywhere within the brain. They can be isolated or multiple. Multiple cavernous angiomas are especially common in familial cases. Familial forms include an autosomal-dominant type, which is present among the American Southwest Hispanic population. The origin of the malformation is uncertain, and new hemorrhagic lesions can appear in a patient with a previously normal MRI. Seizure disorders can occasionally result from cavernous angiomas, and acute hemorrhages can cause focal neurologic symptoms. Despite the tendency for rehemorrhage, many of these lesions are asymptomatic or they cause seizures that can be adequately controlled with medical treatment. Brainstem lesions carry a greater risk from hemorrhage, and larger extra-lesional hemorrhage elsewhere can also cause damage. Larger lesions can also cause some mass effect.

Unlike an AVM, a cavernous angioma is best imaged with MRI. In fact, cavernous angiomas are usually not found on routine angiography. Acute hemorrhage can be observed on CT, and calcification that occurs in a minority of lesions can also be visualized on CT. Some but not all lesions demonstrate contrast enhancement. The classic MRI appearance derives from the multiple ages of blood degradation products present, with a reticulated popcorn- or mulberry-like appearance of mixed methemoglobin and surrounding hemosiderin (Fig. 6–11).

Small lesions often present a target appearance of central bright methemoglobin and a rim of dark hemosiderin on T2-weighted images. A small lesion that has bled may leave only a scar of hemosiderin visible. These smaller lesions are not specific, and similar appearances can be caused by any abnormality that has resulted in a small hemorrhage. A small AVM with slow flow or prior thrombosis may also be angiographically occult and indistinguishable on MRI from a cavernous angioma. Hemorrhagic metastasis may rarely simulate the appearance of a cavernous angioma. Venous angiomas are occasionally associated with a cavernous angioma.

Venous Angioma

Venous angiomas are thought to be developmental variants rather than true vascular malformations. Multiple veins converge to a single draining vein, resulting in a spoke-wheel appearance on imaging. Hemorrhage is infrequent, and some cases of hemorrhage with venous angioma are the result of an associated cavernous angioma. Resection is avoided when possible because the veins provide drainage for functioning brain, and venous infarction can result. The radiating pattern of veins can be seen on the venous phase of angiography, on contrasted CT, or on MRI or MRA (Fig. 6–12).

Other Malformations

Capillary telangiectasias represent a fourth pathologic type of vascular malformation,

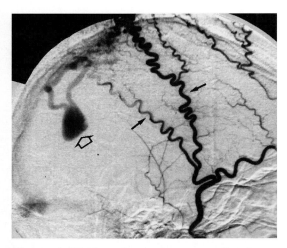

Figure 6–10. Dural arteriovenous fistula. Angiogram, with lateral projection of superficial temporal artery injection. Markedly enlarged and tortuous meningeal arteries *(solid arrows)* lead to abnormally draining veins and a large venous varix *(open arrow)*.

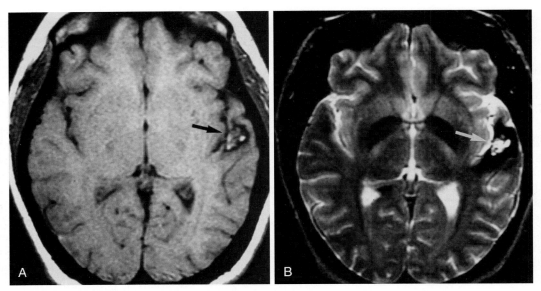

Figure 6–11. Cavernous angioma on MRI. *(A)* Axial T1WI and *(B)* T2WI. There is a heterogeneous signal intensity lesion within the left temporal lobe *(arrows)*. The mixed pattern is consistent with blood products of varying ages, with small, round, bright areas representing methemoglobin and surrounding dark signal intensity, especially on the T2WI, of hemosiderin. Several other cavernous malformations were present elsewhere in the brain in this patient with familial cavernous angiomas.

consisting of dilated capillaries. They rarely bleed and are rarely detected on imaging studies. A small area of enhancement is occasionally observed on contrasted CT or MRI.

The vein of Galen malformation (less ac-

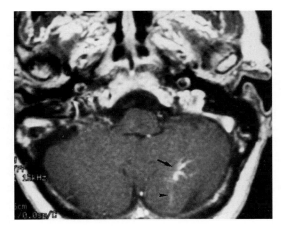

Figure 6–12. Venous angioma. Contrast-enhanced MRI (axial T1WI) shows enhancing veins in the left cerebellar hemisphere in a spokewheel pattern *(arrow)*. The draining vein extends posteriorly *(arrowhead)*.

curately termed a vein of Galen aneurysm) is a congenital vascular malformation that involves an abnormal arterial connection to the deep cerebral venous system. Presenting symptoms can include congestive heart failure, posterior fossa (pineal region) mass, hydrocephalus, and hemorrhage. Typically the vein of Galen is markedly dilated. The dilated vein can be seen with CT or MRI, with the latter having the advantage of multiplanar capability. Full characterization, especially for planning surgical or endovascular therapy, may require angiography.

Carotid-cavernous Fistula

Carotid-cavernous fistulae occur when there is an abnormal connection from the distal internal carotid artery to the cavernous sinus. A direct connection can result from trauma or intracavernous aneurysm. Atherosclerotic disease can also result in an indirect type of connection. The common clinical presentation includes proptosis, chemosis, and orbital bruit. The superior ophthalmic vein is often engorged from retrograde flow. The dilated vein can be seen on

CT or MRI, and MRA can demonstrate the abnormal flow (Fig. 6–13). Endovascular therapy (balloons or coils placed into the cavernous sinus) is often the preferred treatment.

HYPERTENSIVE HEMORRHAGE

After trauma, hypertension is the next most common cause of intracranial hemorrhage in adults. Areas of the brain served by small penetrating arteries, such as the deep gray nuclei, are especially prone to such hemorrhage. The putamen is most commonly affected, followed by the thalamus. The pons and cerebellum near the dentate nuclei are also common sites of hypertensive hemorrhage. Morbidity can be high with large hematomas. Intraventricular extension is relatively common and can lead to hydrocephalus.

The CT appearance is that of acute hemorrhage, with dense blood initially, followed over hours to days by edema and increasing mass effect, then gradual resolution. Hemorrhage in a typical location in a hypertensive patient should suggest the diagnosis (see Fig. 6–2).

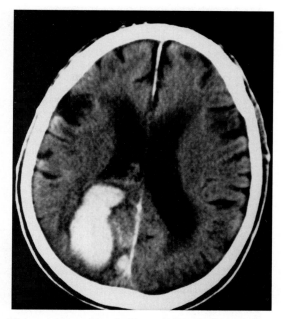

Figure 6–14. Amyloid angiopathy with parenchymal hemorrhage. A large, fairly superficial, intraparenchymal hemorrhage is present in the right parietal lobe in this 90-year-old normotensive man (nonenhanced CT).

OTHER CAUSES OF HEMORRHAGE

The CT finding of lobar hemorrhage in a normotensive, nontraumatized elderly patient should suggest the possibility of amyloid angiopathy (Fig. 6–14). Amyloid angiopathy is a condition in which amyloid protein deposits in the walls of cerebral arterioles predispose to hemorrhage. It affects elderly patients, and multiple episodes of hemorrhage often occur. The location is often subcortical and lobar rather than deep. Hypertensive hemorrhages can occasionally also be peripheral, and thus patient history is essential.

Other vasculopathies can also cause intracranial hemorrhage. A wide variety of causes of vasculitis exist, including infection (meningitis), immune-mediated conditions, radiation, and drugs such as cocaine and methamphetamine. Specific features such as distribution and patterns of arterial change can sometimes suggest an etiology, but in general there is considerable overlap.

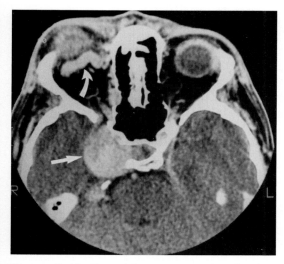

Figure 6–13. Carotid-cavernous fistula. Contrast-enhanced CT scan shows enlarged right cavernous sinus *(straight arrow)*; a tortuous, enlarged right superior ophthalmic vein *(curved arrow)*; and proptosis of the right globe.

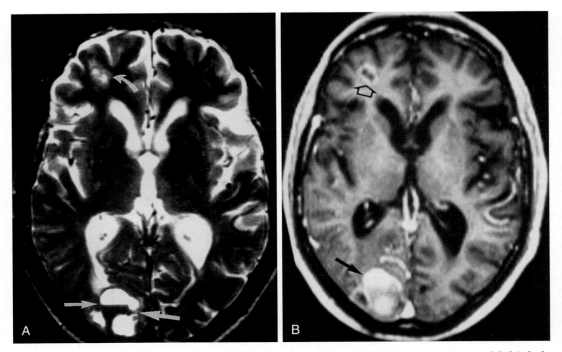

Figure 6–15. Hemorrhagic neoplasm. MRI of a man with metastatic lung carcinoma. Multiple hemorrhagic lesions were present in the brain. *(A)* The axial T2WI shows a complex right posterior cerebral lesion *(straight arrows)* with multiple fluid-fluid layers and areas of different signal intensities. A smaller area of ill-defined high signal intensity is present in the right frontal lobe *(curved arrow).*

(B) After intravenous gadolinium contrast administration (T1WI), a thin rim of enhancement is apparent, but most of the central high signal intensity within the lesion represents methemoglobin *(solid arrow).* Enhancement also occurs around the right frontal metastatic lesion *(open arrow).* The appearance of blood in a hemorrhagic neoplasm is often complex.

Features include arterial narrowing, occlusion, and beading. Hemorrhage and ischemia are possible outcomes. Angiography is the most sensitive imaging test.

Hemorrhagic infarction is discussed in Chapter 5. Premature infants are susceptible to germinal matrix hemorrhage, which is discussed in Chapter 9.

Neoplasms, both primary and metastatic,

can hemorrhage (Chapter 4). Melanoma, renal cell carcinoma, choriocarcinoma, and thyroid metastases are particularly prone to bleeding. Lung and breast carcinoma, because of their frequency, are also among the most common metastatic tumors to hemorrhage. The appearance of blood in hemorrhagic neoplasms is often complex (Fig. 6–15).

Chapter

7

Hydrocephalus

Hydrocephalus refers to ventricular dilatation resulting from excess cerebrospinal fluid (CSF) within the ventricles. In other words, hydrocephalus occurs because of an imbalance between production and resorption of CSF. Both processes are continuous and are normally in equilibrium. In adults, approximately 400 to 500 ml of CSF are produced per day. CSF is secreted by the choroid plexus as an ultrafiltrate of plasma. Most is formed in the lateral ventricles, but choroid plexus tissue is also present in the posterior third and fourth ventricles. CSF normally flows through the ventricular system to the subarachnoid spaces, then over the cerebral convexities, where it is absorbed via the arachnoid villi or granulations in the venous sinuses (Fig. 7–1).

Hydrocephalus is nearly always the result of obstruction of the flow of CSF somewhere along its path from the ventricles to the arachnoid granulations. Overproduction is rarely a cause of hydrocephalus, with the possible exception of choroid plexus papilloma (see Fig. 4–8).

Specific causes of hydrocephalus are discussed in greater detail elsewhere in the book. In this section, general principles relating to hydrocephalus are presented.

HYDROCEPHALUS VERSUS ATROPHY

Not all ventricular dilatation (ventriculomegaly) represents hydrocephalus. Cerebral volume loss can also result in increased ventricular volume, either diffuse or focal. Atrophy must therefore be distinguished from hydrocephalus. Cerebral atrophy results in enlargement of the cortical sulci and basal cisterns. With hydrocephalus, on the other hand, increasing ventricular volume causes mass effect on the surrounding brain, with progressive effacement of sulci. Because of transependymal CSF flow, a rim of edema is often identified surrounding the dilated ventricles. This interstitial edema has intermediate attenuation between that of CSF and brain on CT, and high signal intensity on intermediate- and T2-weighted sequences on MRI.

Normal Pressure Hydrocephalus

Confirming the presence of hydrocephalus can be particularly challenging when cerebral atrophy is also present. The most common circumstance occurs in the elderly patient with normal pressure hydrocephalus (NPH). The pathophysiology of NPH is still in question. Classically, patients present with a clinical triad of dementia, incontinence, and gait apraxia. Measurements of CSF pressure show normal values. Patients with NPH may show improvement with placement of a ventricular shunt.

A degree of cerebral volume loss and some nonspecific periventricular white matter changes on CT, and especially on MRI, are commonly observed with aging. Such invo-

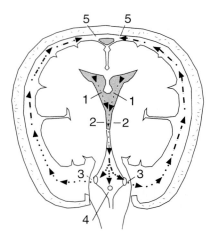

1- Foramina of Monro

2- Aqueduct of Sylvius

3- Foramina of Luschka

4- Foramen of Magendie

5- Arachnoid Granulations

Figure 7–1. CSF flow and potential levels of obstruction to flow. Diagram of the brain and ventricles in coronal section. Arrows indicate the normal direction of CSF flow from its origin in the choroid plexus: from the lateral ventricles through the foramen of Monro (1); through the third ventricle into the cerebral aqueduct (of Sylvius) (2) into the fourth ventricle; through the foramina of Luschka (3) and Magendie (4) into the subarachnoid space; and from the basilar cisterns over the cerebral convexities and to the arachnoid granulations, where it is resorbed. Obstruction anywhere along this pathway may lead to hydrocephalus.

lutional changes correlate only weakly with mental changes in the elderly. Imaging diagnosis of hydrocephalus in older patients depends, therefore, on recognizing disproportionately greater enlargement of the ventricles as compared with the sulci (Fig. 7–2A). On MRI, the periventricular increased signal intensity on T2-weighted images in hydrocephalus is often more smooth and uniform than the periventricular white matter changes of aging. Radionuclide cisternography may be helpful in some cases to confirm abnormal CSF flow (Fig. 7–2B).

LEVELS OF OBSTRUCTION

Obstruction of CSF flow leading to hydrocephalus can occur at several levels, and recognizing the most likely level of obstruction often alters the differential diagnosis (see Fig. 7–1). Although many processes can cause hydrocephalus, some are especially common or have distinctive imaging appearances.

Ventricular Obstruction
Lateral Ventricle Obstruction

Obstruction by a mass within a lateral ventricle causes dilatation of that ventricle only. Common ventricular masses include choroid plexus papillomas, meningiomas, astrocytomas, subependymomas, and ependymomas (Table 7–1). A mass near the foramen of Monro is especially likely to cause obstruction. In addition to the ventricular masses mentioned above, the subependymal giant cell astrocytoma characteristically occurs near the foramen of Monro (see Fig. 9–25). This uncommon, low-grade neoplasm is a significant cause of morbidity in tuberous sclerosis (see Chapter 9). Masses at the foramen of Monro may cause obstruction and enlargement of both lateral ventricles.

Third Ventricle Obstruction

Third ventricular masses lead to obstruction of both lateral ventricles. Anterior masses block the foramen of Monro. In this case, the third ventricle itself may or may not be dilated. A common anterior third ventricle mass is the colloid cyst. Colloid cysts are developmental, probably of endodermal origin, although other theories have been proposed. Gelatinous fluid forms from the lining, and the cyst gradually enlarges. Headache caused by obstruction is the most common clinical manifestation. There may be a positional component, with symptoms

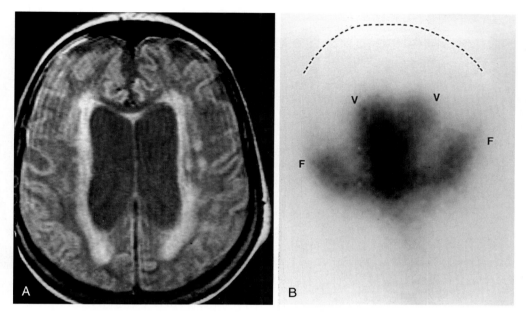

Figure 7–2. Normal pressure hydrocephalus (NPH). *(A)* MRI (axial intermediate-weighted image) of a 70-year-old patient with clinical signs consistent with NPH shows enlarged ventricles (disproportionate to sulcal enlargement), with a rim of periventricular increased signal intensity (transependymal flow of CSF). A radionuclide cisternogram using indium-111 was performed. *(B)* Anteroposterior view 24 hours following intrathecal injection shows activity within the lateral ventricles (V) and sylvian fissures (F) but no activity over the convexities (dotted lines indicate convexities). A similar pattern remained at 48 and 72 hours after infection. Activity normally is present over the convexities by 24 hours and is absent within the ventricles.

alleviated as the cyst moves away from the foramen (ball-valve effect). Sudden death resulting from obstruction has been reported on rare occasions. The imaging appearance is that of a round, midline mass in the anterior third ventricle (Fig. 7–3).

TABLE 7–1. **Lateral Ventricle Masses**

Children
　Astrocytoma
　Primitive neuroectodermal tumor (PNET)
　Choroid plexus papilloma
　Giant cell astrocytoma (children and young
　　adults with tuberous sclerosis)
　Ependymoma
Adults
　Meningioma
　Astrocytoma
　Oligodendroglioma
　Central neurocytoma
　Subependymoma
　Metastasis

Because the fluid within the cyst is quite variable in both viscosity and content, the density and signal intensity are also variable. If intravenous contrast material is given, the rim occasionally enhances, but the contents do not.

Posterior third ventricle masses may be difficult to differentiate on CT from pineal region and tectal region masses. Meningioma, choroid plexus papilloma, and metastases are the most common tumors that occur in this location. The multiplanar capability of MRI is helpful in evaluating this region (Fig. 7–4). The third and lateral ventricles are dilated, whereas the fourth ventricle remains normal in size.

Pineal Region and Aqueductal Obstruction

Masses of the pineal gland itself or masses near the pineal gland cause compression of the tectum and obstruction of the cerebral aqueduct. Third and lateral ventricle dilata-

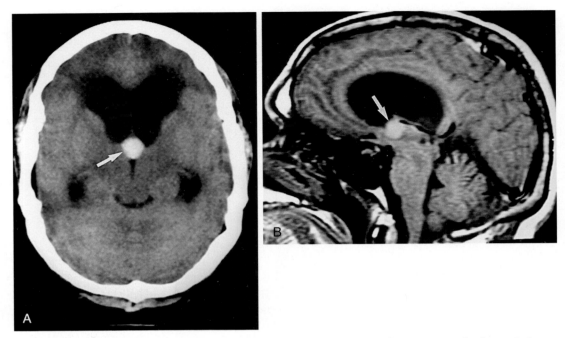

Figure 7–3. Colloid cyst. *(A)* Noncontrast CT of a 49-year-old man demonstrates hydrocephalus and a dense cyst *(arrow)* at the foramen of Monro. *(B)* On MRI (sagittal T1WI) the cyst *(arrow)* has mildly increased signal intensity relative to brain.

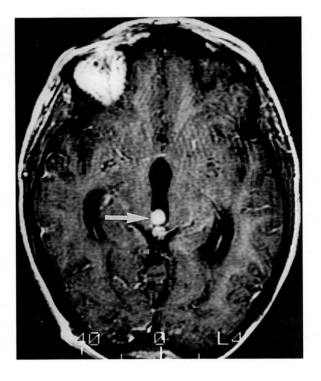

Figure 7–4. Posterior third ventricle mass. Axial MRI (T1WI after gadolinium administration) of a young woman with headaches shows an enhancing posterior third ventricle mass (ependymoma, *arrow*). The third ventricle and temporal horns of the lateral ventricles are dilated. The fourth ventricle, not pictured, is normal in size. (White area in the upper left of the image is fat within the right orbit.)

TABLE 7–2. Pineal Region Masses

Pineal cell tumors
  Pineoblastoma
  Pineocytoma
Germ cell tumors
  Germinoma
  Teratoma
  Dermoid
  Other
Other tumors (originating in adjacent structures)
  Meningioma
  Astrocytoma (thalamus, tectum, corpus callosum)
  Metastasis
  Vascular malformation

tion results. Paralysis of upward gaze (Parinaud's syndrome) is the classic presentation of pineal region masses that compress the superior colliculi of the tectum. MRI is the imaging test of choice for this region. Masses of this region are listed in Table 7–2.

Other causes of obstruction at the level of the cerebral aqueduct include tectal gliomas or astrocytomas and aqueductal stenosis. Intrinsic midbrain neoplasms are recognized more readily with MRI than with CT. Depending on their size and caudal extent, they can spare or deform the fourth ventri-

cle, but the fourth ventricle is usually not enlarged.

Aqueductal stenosis often presents clinically in infancy. However, stenosis without complete obstruction of the aqueduct can result in a mild compensated enlargement of the ventricular system (third and lateral ventricles) that may not become symptomatic for many years. In addition to the expected changes in ventricular configuration, narrowing of the aqueduct itself can occasionally be observed on high-resolution sagittal MRI (Fig. 7–5).

Posterior Fossa Masses

In adults, metastatic neoplasms are the most common posterior fossa masses. The histologic spectrum of posterior fossa masses in children is quite different. Posterior fossa masses are a significant cause of morbidity and death in childhood. Although the overall frequency of such neoplasms is low, CNS tumors are the second most common type of childhood tumor, and posterior fossa masses constitute a major fraction of childhood brain tumors. Clinical manifestations include those resulting from hydrocephalus (see Figs. 4–5, 4–7), ataxia and other cerebellar symptoms, and cranial nerve and brainstem symptoms. Posterior

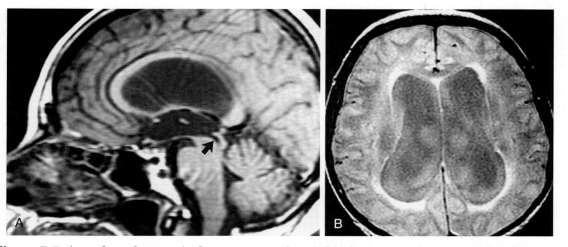

Figure 7–5. Aqueductal stenosis, late presentation. MRI of a woman who presented with headaches. *(A)* Sagittal T1WI shows prominence of the proximal cerebral aqueduct *(arrow)*. The caudal portion of the aqueduct is stenotic. The corpus callosum is thinned. *(B)* Axial intermediate-weighted (long TR/short TE) image shows enlarged lateral ventricles. A thin rim of periventricular increased signal intensity represents transependymal CSF flow (interstitial edema).

fossa masses are listed in Table 7–3, and brain neoplasms are discussed in greater detail in Chapter 4.

Medulloblastomas, or primitive neuroectodermal tumors (PNET) of the posterior fossa, represent about 30 to 40 percent of posterior fossa masses in children. The most common location is in the midline, near the floor of the fourth ventricle, but they can also occur in the cerebellar hemisphere. They often have relatively high attenuation on CT, usually higher than that of normal brain tissue.

Cerebellar astrocytomas constitute a slightly smaller fraction of childhood posterior fossa masses. Most are of the pilocytic type, which generally has a very good prognosis. Cysts, often associated with mural nodules, are commonly present within the tumor. On CT, astrocytomas are usually less dense than brain.

Brainstem gliomas are infiltrative and demonstrate variable enhancement.

Ependymomas are the fourth most common childhood posterior fossa mass. They are usually intraventricular, most commonly involving the fourth ventricle and

having a marked propensity for extension through the foramina into adjacent subarachnoid cisterns. Ependymomas often spread throughout the subarachnoid spaces via the CSF.

Congenital Posterior Fossa Anomalies

The Chiari II malformation is nearly always associated with some degree of obstruction to ventricular flow (see Fig. 9–4). Although various abnormalities of the ventricular system occur, including aqueductal obstruction, the fourth ventricle is nearly always small and low. Ventricular shunting procedures are usually necessary. The Chiari I malformation is less often associated with hydrocephalus. Chapter 9 provides more detailed discussion of these congenital hindbrain malformations, as well as the Dandy-Walker malformation (see Fig. 9–6).

Extraventricular Obstruction (Communicating Hydrocephalus)

Outside the ventricular system, obstruction to CSF flow can occur at the level of the basilar cisterns. Central nervous system tuberculosis is a classic cause of basilar meningitis (see Fig. 3–7), but fungal infections (coccidioidomycosis and cryptococcosis), cysticercosis, and sarcoidosis are also associated with basilar cistern disease that can lead to obstruction (see Fig. 3–10B). Contrast enhancement is often necessary to identify inflammatory processes around the base of the brain (see Chapter 3). Meningeal carcinomatosis can also cause enhancement of the meninges.

Several processes can lead to blockage of CSF resorption at the level of the arachnoid granulations, especially subarachnoid hemorrhage and infection. A previous episode of meningitis or hemorrhage often results in a communicating type of hydrocephalus, one of the most common forms of hydrocephalus (see Figs. 3–2, 3–11). The entire ventricular system is usually enlarged if the level of obstruction is outside the ventricles (i.e., anywhere from the outlets of the fourth ventricle, to the basilar cisterns, to the arachnoid granulations). However, the third and lateral ventricles usually dilate before the

---

TABLE 7–3. **Posterior Fossa Masses**

Intra-axial or Ventricular
Children
Medulloblastoma (small, round cell tumors, dense on CT)
Astrocytoma (usually juvenile pilocytic variety, low density on CT)
Brainstem glioma (infiltrative)
Ependymoma of the fourth ventricle (often extrude through foramina)
Adults
Metastases (most common)
Hemangioblastoma (uncommon)
Choroid plexus papilloma (rare)
Subependymoma (usually incidental, rarely symptomatic)

Extra-axial
Inflammatory cysts (e.g., cysticercosis)
Cerebellopontine angle masses
Schwannoma
Meningioma
Epidermoid
Other (see Table 4–3)

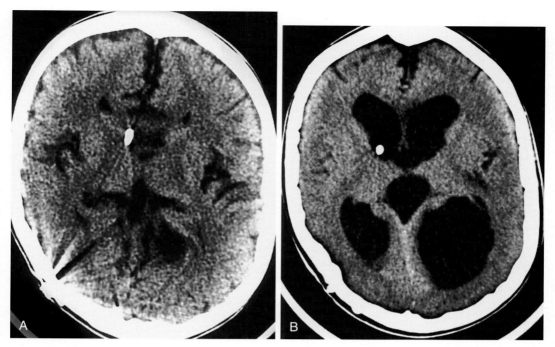

Figure 7–6. Shunt failure. *(A)* The ventricles are small on early CT scan of the brain of a child with Chiari II malformation. The shunt catheter tip and artifact from the shunt reservoir are visible. *(B)* CT scan obtained when the child returned with vomiting shows severe interval dilatation of the third and lateral ventricles.

fourth, so determining an exact level of obstruction may not always be possible.

IMAGING FOLLOWING THE TREATMENT OF HYDROCEPHALUS

Imaging is important for the evaluation of the treatment of hydrocephalus. Following the performance of a ventricular shunt procedure, the brain and ventricles may take some time to return to a more normal configuration, especially if hydrocephalus has been long-standing. CT is the most commonly used imaging method for following a patient with a ventricular shunt, although MRI can also be useful. Clinical suspicion of shunt malfunction is an indication for follow-up scans. If a catheter is no longer functioning properly, the ventricles increase in size (Fig. 7–6).

8

Multiple Sclerosis and Degenerative Diseases of the Brain

Neurodegenerative diseases are a diverse group of disorders that adversely affect many patients, especially the elderly. However, multiple sclerosis (MS) is a major cause of disability in young and middle-aged adults. Neurodegenerative diseases are uncommon in childhood but may have devastating consequences. Typical clinical manifestations include dementia, movement disorders, weakness and sensory loss, and, in children, loss of developmental milestones.

This chapter includes a discussion of MS, white matter diseases that may have a similar appearance to MS, dysmyelinating and other degenerative diseases of childhood, changes of aging, common diseases that result in dementia and movement abnormalities, and some reversible conditions of vascular origin. Imaging can be very helpful in the diagnosis of some of these diseases. Imaging is also occasionally useful in monitoring therapy. In the evaluation of such common disorders as dementia, the primary role of imaging is to aid in the detection of the subgroup of treatable conditions. Because CT and MRI findings alone are seldom specific in this group of diseases, these studies must be interpreted in the setting of relevant clinical information.

MULTIPLE SCLEROSIS AND OTHER DEMYELINATING DISEASES

MS is an inflammatory demyelinating disease of the brain and spinal cord of uncertain etiology. The disease is immune-mediated, with complex genetic and environmental susceptibilities. Pathologically, perivenular inflammation is observed, with subsequent destruction of myelin and the formation of plaques. Early inflammatory changes may relapse and remit, but recurrent demyelination leads to gliosis (scarring) and loss of axons.

Clinical Features and Treatment

Multiple clinical episodes occurring over time, with varying neurologic deficits, are the hallmark of the disease. Women are affected more often than men by approximately a two-to-one ratio, with peak onset in young adulthood to middle age. MS in children is rare but can occur. Geographic differences in incidence also occur, with much less MS in tropical regions than in northern latitudes. Optic neuritis is a frequent manifestation (Fig. 8–1). The spinal cord is often involved. Sensory loss, weak-

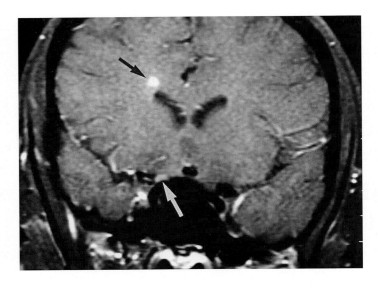

Figure 8–1. Optic neuritis and multiple sclerosis. MRI (gadolinium-enhanced coronal T1WI with fat suppression) of a 28-year-old woman with sudden right eye visual loss. The right optic nerve enhances *(white arrow)*. Two periventricular plaques were present on T2WI, one of which also enhances *(black arrow)*.

ness, visual impairment, and bladder dysfunction are common.

Although a waxing and waning course with remission of symptoms is typical, the course of a subgroup of patients may demonstrate progressive and unremitting deterioration. For decades, treatment was largely supportive. However, research has identified medications that are beneficial for some patients.

Diagnosis of MS

The diagnosis of MS rests on historic and clinical findings and supporting laboratory and imaging test results. No definitive laboratory test exists for MS. Oligoclonal bands in the CSF are often present but constitute a nonspecific finding. Early in the course of MS, imaging abnormalities may be mild or absent. However, with progression of the disease, scans are often strikingly abnormal. Although nonspecific, MRI abnormalities may strongly suggest MS. With increasingly effective therapy, MRI may be helpful as an aid to monitoring treatment.

Imaging in MS

MRI is the imaging technique of choice for MS. Although MS plaques may appear as areas of low density on CT, MRI is far more sensitive (Fig. 8–2). Multiple sclerosis plaques appear as areas of high signal in-

tensity on both intermediate and T2-weighted images (first- and second-echo, long TR spin-echo images). Periventricular lesions are common, and plaques can be difficult to distinguish from adjacent CSF on heavily T2-weighted images. Sequences in which plaques remain bright but CSF is darker therefore are more useful. These include intermediate-weighted (short TE/long TR) spin-echo sequences (Fig. 8–3A,B) and inversion recovery sequences designed to attenuate fluid signal. The plaques appear round to oval, and the long axis of oval lesions is sometimes oriented perpendicular to the long axis of the ventricles. As the demyelination process proceeds, the areas of abnormal signal intensity on MRI can become confluent.

In addition to periventricular lesions, subcortical, brainstem, and cerebellar lesions may occur (Fig. 8–3C). The corpus callosum is often involved, and lesions along the inferior margin of the corpus callosum, or callosal-septal interface, especially suggest MS (Fig. 8–3D). The basal ganglia can be affected, despite being primarily composed of gray matter. With axonal loss, volume loss occurs, and areas of encephalomalacia appear as low signal intensity on T1-weighted images. Callosal atrophy and diffuse cortical atrophy ensue.

Much of the symptomatology of MS results from lesions not in the brain but in the

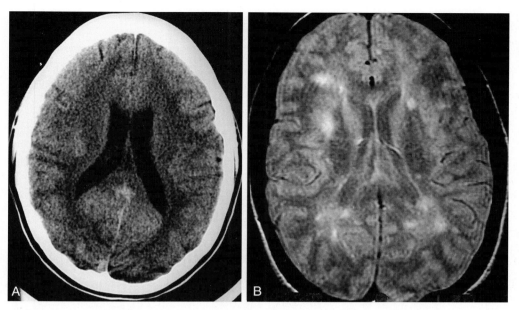

Figure 8–2. Multiple sclerosis (MS), CT versus MRI. *(A)* Nonenhanced CT scan is normal. Following contrast administration, a single small focus of enhancement was observed. *(B)* MRI obtained 1 day later (axial intermediate-weighted image) reveals numerous areas of increased signal intensity in MS plaques. Several plaques enhanced following gadolinium administration. MRI is the imaging test of choice for MS.

spinal cord. These symptoms include patchy numbness, spastic weakness, and bladder and gait dysfunction.

During the active inflammatory phase, solid or ring-like contrast enhancement of plaques can be seen. The differential diagnosis of ring-enhancing lesions of the brain also includes primary and metastatic neoplasms, abscess, and resolving infarctions and hematomas. Although enhancement presumably indicates active inflammation, the correlation of enhancing brain plaques with clinical symptoms is weak. Brain MRI shows that MS is a dynamic disease, with plaques appearing and disappearing in the absence of clinical symptoms. A large mass with enhancement and edema is an uncommon presentation of MS.

DIFFERENTIAL DIAGNOSIS OF WHITE MATTER DISEASE

In addition to MS, the differential diagnosis of multiple white matter lesions includes a wide variety of processes that lead to edema, gliosis, or demyelination. Processes such as hypertension, migraine headaches, and vasculitis lead to small vessel disease and can cause scattered white matter changes on MRI. Neoplasms, particularly metastatic disease, can cause multiple focal areas of increased signal intensity on T2-weighted MRI, but some mass effect is often, although not invariably, present. Parenchymal infections may cause focal white matter abnormalities on MRI. Primary HIV infection can cause scattered or confluent white matter changes. Central nervous system Lyme disease has been described as sometimes causing white matter changes that resemble MS. Acute disseminated encephalitis or encephalomyelitis (ADEM) is an inflammatory process that typically occurs several weeks after a viral infection or vaccination. Scattered areas of abnormal signal intensity are present, usually in a subcortical distribution. Contrast enhancement can occur. In some cases, ADEM can be distinguished from an initial attack of MS only when MRI changes or symptoms recur with MS.

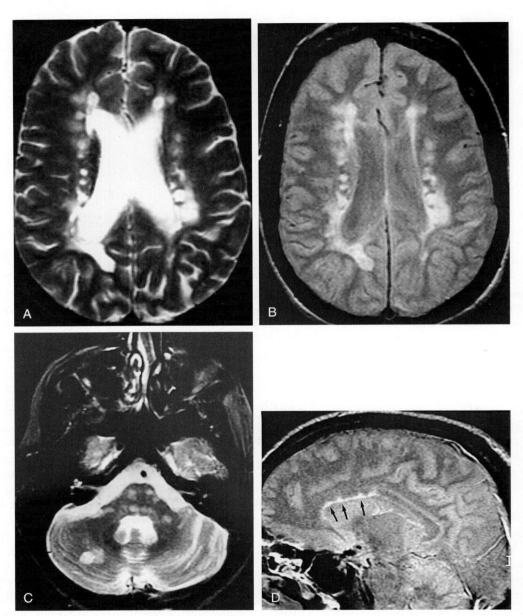

Figure 8–3. Multiple sclerosis. MRI of a 46-year-old woman with clinical criteria of MS. *(A)* Axial T2WI through the level of the bodies of the lateral ventricles shows numerous periventricular areas of increased signal intensity compatible with plaques of MS. *(B)* Extent of periventricular involvement is easier to visualize on the intermediate-weighted (long TR/short TE) image (first echo from the same sequence) at the same level. CSF fades to intermediate signal intensity on this image, whereas areas of edema and demyelination remain bright. *(C)* Axial T2WI at the level of the fourth ventricle demonstrates plaques in the pons, middle cerebellar peduncles, and cerebellum. *(D)* Sagittal intermediate-weighted image of another patient shows several lesions *(arrows,* high signal intensity) along the inferior margin of the corpus callosum, a location strongly suggestive of MS.

DYSMYELINATING DISEASES AND DEPOSITION DISEASES

Various inborn errors of metabolism can cause defects in the normal myelination process. They are uncommon conditions, but the imaging appearance may be striking.

Adrenoleukodystrophy (ALD) is an X-linked condition that usually presents in the first decade of life. Cerebral and spinal cord deterioration follow. Adrenal insufficiency, when it occurs, often follows neurologic deterioration. The diagnosis is made by assays of plasma, erythrocytes, or cultured skin fibroblasts for very-long-chain fatty acids that accumulate as a result of a peroxisomal abnormality. Cranial MRI shows symmetric, confluent high signal intensity on T2-weighted images that begins in the occipital white matter and advances frontally over time (Fig. 8–4). Noncontrasted CT shows low attenuation in a corresponding distribution. If intravenous contrast material is administered, the anterior margin of the demyelination may enhance.

Metachromatic leukodystrophy is the

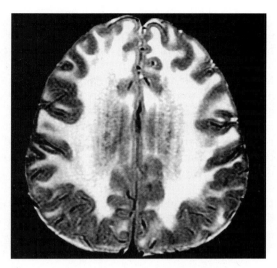

Figure 8–5. Leukoencephalopathy, probable Canavan's disease. MRI of a 3-year-old with developmental delay and large head circumference. Severe leukoencephalopathy is manifested by high signal intensity in all cerebral white matter on the axial T2WI.

most common inherited leukodystrophy. It is caused by diminished amounts or decreased function of arylsulfatase A. Abnormal myelination results in progressive deterioration of central nervous system function and death. The peripheral nervous system myelin is also involved. Various forms have been described, and the age of presentation varies. Most patients present in childhood. CT and MRI show diffuse abnormal attenuation or signal intensity, respectively, in the deep cerebral white matter, as well as atrophy.

Alexander's disease and Canavan's disease are leukodystrophies in which the head circumference is increased. Cerebral white matter shows abnormal attenuation or signal intensity on CT or MRI (Fig. 8–5). Initially the peripheral white matter is most involved, although more diffuse disease is observed over time. The white matter changes in Alexander's disease begin in the frontal lobes and move posteriorly.

Defects in mitochondrial function cause Leigh disease and other diseases classified as mitochondrial disorders. The lentiform nuclei and thalami are often affected in these diseases.

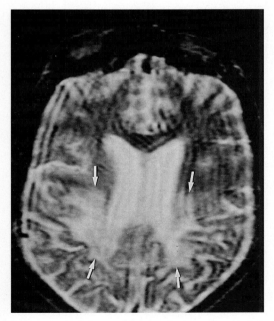

Figure 8–4. Adrenal leukodystrophy. Axial T2WI from MRI of a 13-year-old boy demonstrates confluent high signal intensity in the posterior white matter *(arrows),* as well as atrophy.

A wide range of uncommon deposition diseases and enzyme defects can result in cerebral degeneration visible on neuroimaging studies. In some instances, more specific features can be helpful, such as high attenuation in the thalami on CT in Krabbe's disease or lack of brain myelination in Pelizaeus-Merzbacher disease. Biochemical test results are usually essential in diagnosis of these conditions, although the combination of clinical presentation and imaging test results can suggest the diagnosis. Imaging of these uncommon diseases is discussed in detail in textbooks of pediatric neuroradiology.

AGING, DEMENTIA, AND NEURODEGENERATIVE DISEASES

Changes of Aging

In evaluating the aging brain, it is important to recognize the common changes observed in healthy elderly patients. These changes can occasionally be extensive, with considerable overlap with pathologic processes. Some degree of parenchymal volume loss is the rule with increasing age. Atrophy alone is therefore not necessarily pathologic in elderly patients. Areas of white matter hyperintensity are seen with increasing frequency in later decades. These can be in the periventricular white matter and centrum semiovale, as well as in the subcortical white matter (Fig. 8–6). White matter changes of aging do not exhibit mass effect or contrast enhancement. Periventricular changes can become confluent. Various explanations of these tissue changes have been proposed. It is likely that several mechanisms create these areas of increased signal intensity on MRI.

Extensive white matter changes in young or middle-aged patients are not normal, but the significance of these MRI findings is problematic in elderly patients. Although white matter hyperintensities may be observed in multi-infarct dementia and other pathologic states, the appearance is so common in the aging brain that it has poor specificity. For example, there is very little correlation between mental function and the extent of white matter changes in elderly patients. Given this poor correlation, one of the main goals of MRI in elderly patients with mental status changes is to detect treatable conditions, such as hydrocephalus or subdural hematoma, not to look for white matter changes or atrophy.

Dementia and Movement Disorders

Although there are limitations in interpreting involutional changes, some neurodegenerative processes have distinctive imaging features that can aid in their diagnosis.

Alzheimer's disease is a common cause of dementia. Atrophy is seen on CT and MRI, especially in the region of the hippocampus and the remainder of the temporal lobes. Parietal and frontal atrophy also follow. White matter disease is not a diagnostic feature of Alzheimer's disease. Positron emission tomography (PET) or single-pho-

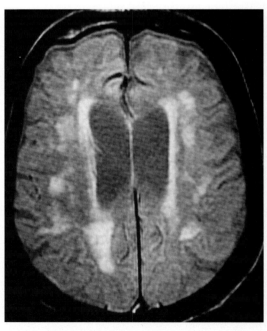

Figure 8–6. Aging brain. MRI (intermediate-weighted, or long TR/short TE) of an asymptomatic, healthy 88-year-old man. The ventricles and sulci are enlarged. Scattered areas of increased signal intensity in periventricular and subcortical white matter are common with aging and do not represent areas of infarction.

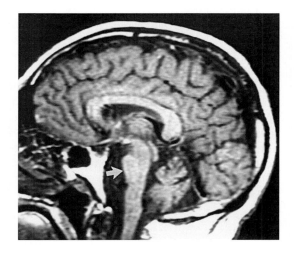

Figure 8–7. Olivopontocerebellar degeneration. MRI (sagittal T1WI) of a man with progressive ataxia shows atrophy of the cerebellum and pons. Much less atrophy was present on an earlier scan. The prepontine cistern is enlarged because of pontine degeneration. The anterior margin of the pons is flattened *(arrow)* because of atrophy.

ton emission CT (SPECT) studies of metabolism or blood flow show diminished function of the parietal and temporal lobes. Pick's disease (frontotemporal dementia) is another much less common cause of cortical dementia. Lobar atrophy, especially that involving the frontal lobes, is a feature of this disease.

Subcortical neurodegenerative processes include idiopathic Parkinson's disease and other parkinsonian conditions. Movement disorders are a prominent clinical feature of these diseases. Degeneration of the striatonigral pathways can sometimes be observed on MRI as decreased size of the pars compacta of the substantia nigra. Increasing iron deposition in the globus pallidus, substantia nigra, red nucleus, and dentate

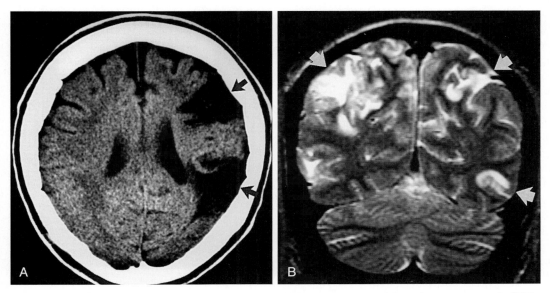

Figure 8–8. Imaging appearance in the brain with SLE. *(A)* Axial CT of a woman with SLE shows infarctions in the left frontal and parietal lobes *(arrows).* Infarctions are especially common in patients with antiphospholipid antibody. *(B)* MRI (coronal T2WI) of a patient with lupus cerebritis shows multiple subcortical and cortical areas of edema *(arrows).* Unlike the infarctions shown in *A,* these changes are reversible. Such findings in SLE may in part be due to hypertensive encephalopathy.

nucleus is normal with aging, and is manifested by low signal intensity on T2-weighted MRI. However, abnormalities of iron deposition can accompany some movement disorders. Increased iron deposition can also be observed with MS. A similar appearance occurs in some chronic intoxications, such as toluene abuse. Patterns of nuclei involved can provide supportive diagnostic evidence but are not pathognomonic.

Cerebellar Atrophy

Various processes can cause atrophy of the cerebellum. Toxic causes include ethanol abuse and long-term phenytoin use. Paraneoplastic syndromes causing cerebellar degeneration may occur with lung, uterine, or ovarian cancer. Degenerative conditions, such as olivopontocerebellar degeneration (OPCD), cause atrophy that is visible on MRI in specific locations (small medullary olives, atrophy of the cerebellum, and flattening of the pons in OPCD; Fig. 8–7).

Huntington's Disease

Several genetic diseases cause distinctive findings on MRI. Huntington's disease is an autosomal dominant condition that causes choreoathetoid movements and progressive dementia. Volume loss in the basal ganglia, especially atrophy of the caudate heads, may be observed on MRI or CT.

Reversible Changes of Vascular Origin

Reversible changes can occur in some diseases of inflammatory or vascular origin. Cerebral changes are not uncommon in systemic lupus erythematosus (SLE). Large or medium vessel infarction can occasionally occur (Fig. 8–8*A*). However, smaller areas of cortical and subcortical increased T2-weighted signal intensity are common in lupus cerebritis (Fig. 8–8*B*). Diffuse volume loss may be observed with high-dose steroid administration but also occurs as a sequela of prolonged disease.

Hypertensive encephalopathy is another possible cause of cortical and subcortical increased signal intensity on T2-weighted scans. The occipital lobes are common sites of abnormality in various hypertensive emergencies, including eclampsia and preeclampsia as well as SLE and other medical causes of hypertension. Other lobes and the basal ganglia may also be involved. These changes usually resolve when the hypertension resolves or is treated.

Chapter

9

Pediatric Neuroradiology

CONSIDERATIONS IN NEUROIMAGING OF CHILDREN

In nearly every category of disease, pediatric neuroradiology involves significant differences from adult neuroradiology. Differences include relative incidences of diseases, types of diseases, and clinical manifestations. Many imaging abnormalities that are similar in both children and adults are presented in other chapters of this book. The focus in this section is on conditions that pertain primarily, if not uniquely, to children.

The choice of which imaging modality to use in children varies with the clinical setting. Cranial ultrasound technique can be performed on infants with an open fontanelle. It is relatively inexpensive and can be obtained at the bedside. However, it is also highly operator-dependent. As with adults, CT is often the study of choice when acute intracranial hemorrhage is suspected (after infancy). MRI is a particularly attractive choice in children for many diagnostic conditions. It avoids ionizing radiation and is superior to CT in discriminating many soft tissue differences. The largest drawback to MRI in children is the longer imaging times required. Improvements in software and newer pulse sequences continue to shorten imaging times.

For young children, sedation is often necessary in both MRI and CT if motion artifacts are to be avoided. Protocols should be

established at each imaging site for pediatric sedation, addressing such issues as parental education, patient preparation, drugs and dosages to be employed, monitoring procedures, and recovery.

CONGENITAL BRAIN MALFORMATIONS

Both CT and MRI reveal major features of congenital brain abnormalities, but MRI has the benefit of being able to readily create images in multiple planes. Sagittal and coronal images are often advantageous in depicting some congenital anomalies. The greater sensitivity of MRI to soft tissue differences makes it much easier to see gray and white matter abnormalities such as neuronal migration anomalies.

Cephaloceles

A cephalocele is a protrusion of cranial contents through a defect in the skull. Cephaloceles are named for the location of the skull defect. The term *encephalocele* is used if brain tissues as well as meninges are included in the protrusion.

Congenital cephaloceles are anomalies of neural tube closure. Marked regional and ethnic variations of incidence occur. Occipital cephaloceles are most common in North America (Fig. 9–1), whereas nasal/ethmoi-

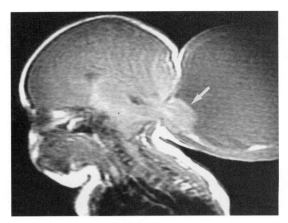

Figure 9–1. Cephalocele, Chiari III. MRI (sagittal T1WI) of a newborn. There is a huge fluid-filled sac at the occiput. Some cerebellar tissue also herniates into the encephalocele *(arrow).*

dal cephaloceles are more common in Asia. Parietal and frontal lesions are relatively uncommon. Sphenoidal cephaloceles may be occult for some time, because the defect is not immediately obvious, as it is in other locations. As with spinal dysraphism, cranial meningeal protrusions may contain neural tissue. Such tissue is usually dysfunctional, but MRI is helpful in evaluating the contents of the cephalocele and its relation to remaining brain.

Chiari Malformations

Chiari malformations are a group of disorders of the posterior fossa. Chiari I malformation is manifested by extension of the cerebellar tonsils inferior to the foramen magnum (Fig. 9–2A). Extension of the cerebellar tonsils several millimeters below the foramen magnum is common and normal. However, a 5-mm or greater extension of the tonsils below the foramen magnum is often associated with symptoms and is considered to be consistent with the designation of Chiari I malformation. No precise numeric definition exists for abnormal tonsillar position, and widespread use of MRI has made it clear that minor degrees of tonsillar extension below the foramen magnum are common. The symptoms of Chiari I malformation are often related to hydrocephalus and/or syrinx, which are commonly associated with this malformation (Fig. 9–2B). Cranial nerve symptoms may also occur.

The Chiari II (Arnold-Chiari) malforma-

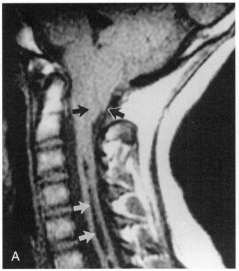
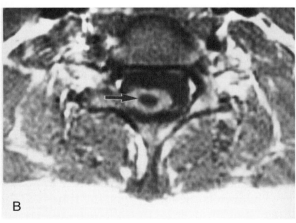

Figure 9–2. Chiari I, syrinx. MRI of the spine was performed in this teenager with atypical scoliosis. *(A)* Sagittal T1WI shows the cerebellar tonsils *(black arrows)* extending more than 2 cm below the foramen magnum, severely narrowing the usual space around the upper spinal cord. Low intensity fluid *(white arrows)* is present within the mid- to lower cervical spinal cord. *(B)* Presence of a syrinx is also confirmed on axial T1WI as central fluid within the spinal cord *(arrow).*

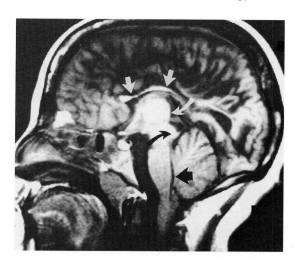

Figure 9–3. Chiari II malformation. MRI of a 14-year-old girl with spina bifida. Sagittal T1WI shows small posterior fossa; "beaked" tectum *(curved black arrow)*; large massa intermedia *(curved white arrow)*; towering cerebellum; small, low fourth ventricle *(straight black arrow)*; and dysgenetic (small and incomplete) corpus callosum *(straight white arrows)*.

tion is a distinctive entity strongly associated with spinal myelomeningocele. It is characterized by a small posterior fossa and a low small fourth ventricle (Figs. 9–3, 9–4). Numerous associated imaging abnormalities are variably present. These include posterior "beaking" of the tectum; a "towering" cerebellum extending rostrally through the tentorial notch; dysgenesis of the corpus callosum; fenestration of the falx cerebri with interdigitation of the hemispheres across the midline; scalloping of the bones consti-

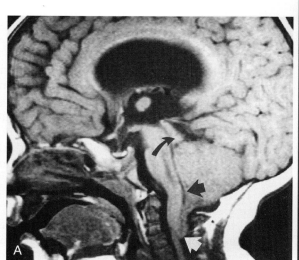

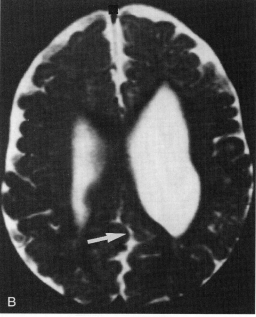

Figure 9–4. Chiari II malformation. MRI of a 1-year-old with spina bifida and repaired lumbar myelomeningocele. *(A)* Sagittal T1WI shows a small posterior fossa; small, low fourth ventricle, which is almost slit-like *(straight black arrow)*; distorted tectum *(curved black arrow)*; and downward cerebellar displacement into the upper cervical spinal canal, with cervicomedullary kinking *(white arrow)*. The corpus callosum is elevated because of hydrocephalus. *(B)* Axial T2WI shows enlarged ventricles and interdigitation of medial cortical gyri across the midline *(arrow)*.

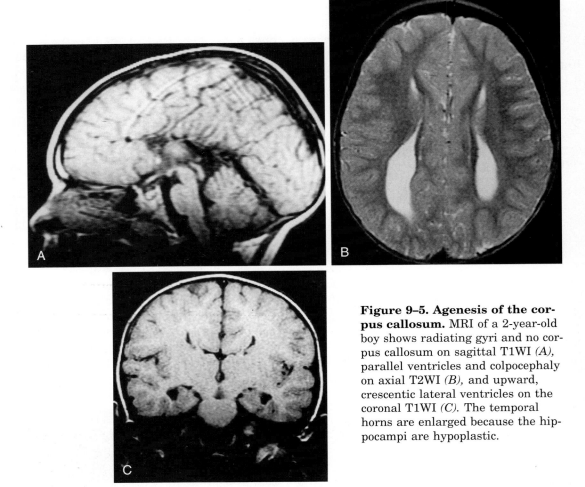

Figure 9–5. Agenesis of the corpus callosum. MRI of a 2-year-old boy shows radiating gyri and no corpus callosum on sagittal T1WI *(A),* parallel ventricles and colpocephaly on axial T2WI *(B),* and upward, crescentic lateral ventricles on the coronal T1WI *(C).* The temporal horns are enlarged because the hippocampi are hypoplastic.

tuting the posterior fossa; and dysplasia of membranous bone (lückenschädel or craniolacunia) producing indentations on the inner surface of the skull during the first year of life. Hydrocephalus is usually present (see Fig. 9–4). Because of the presence of a meningocele or myelomeningocele, the condition is generally detected very early in life.

Chiari III malformation, which is rare, consists of cranial features of Chiari II malformation combined with an encephalocele (see Fig. 9–1).

Disorders of the Corpus Callosum

Disorders of the corpus callosum range from complete absence (agenesis) to mild hypogenesis. The corpus callosum generally develops from the region of the genu posteriorly to the splenium, with the rostrum forming last. Predictably, only the earliest portion of the corpus callosum to form may be present in hypogenesis. Lesions that secondarily destroy portions of the corpus callosum, such as ischemic or infectious damage, do not follow this pattern.

In the absence of the corpus callosum, a characteristic appearance is seen (Fig. 9–5). The lateral ventricles have a more parallel configuration, and the posterior portions demonstrate colpocephaly, that is, enlargement of the posterior body of the lateral ventricles, occipital horns, and atria. The frontal horns demonstrate an upward crescentic appearance. An interhemispheric cyst is often present. The anterior cerebral artery lacks its usual anterior curve, because it can extend straight up rather than wrapping around the genu of the corpus callosum. Sagittal images on MRI illustrate a radial pattern of the medial gyri of the cerebral hemispheres. Colpocephaly and straight ventricles may be the most prominent features when hypogenesis exists. Callosal agenesis alone may be accompanied by few or no symptoms, but it is often associated with many other midline congenital anomalies of the brain (Fig. 9–6).

Lipomas of the corpus callosum are fairly common and are associated with callosal dysgenesis. Fat is readily and specifically identified with either CT or MRI (Fig. 9–7). Lipomas may extend around or adjacent to the corpus callosum. Lipomas may also occur elsewhere in the subarachnoid space around the brain and probably represent abnormal development rather than true neoplasms. Calcification is common.

Holoprosencephalies and Septo-optic Dysplasia

Incomplete or abnormal cleavage of the structures of the forebrain results in holo-prosencephaly (Fig. 9–8). Holoprosencephaly is characterized by lack of complete midline separation of the hemispheres and diencephalon. The condition includes a wide spectrum of abnormalities, with more severe abnormalities on imaging accompanying a worse clinical prognosis. Severe midline facial anomalies are usually present with alobar holoprosencephaly, the most severe form. A single holoventricle is present instead of separate lateral ventricles, the thalami are fused, and the falx cerebri is absent. More separation of midline structures is present in semilobar holoprosencephaly, and lobar holoprosencephaly is the least severe form.

Septo-optic dysplasia, in which there is congenital absence of the septum pellucidum and hypoplasia of optic nerves, may be at the mildest end of this spectrum. A second etiology of septo-optic dysplasia is related to an early injury causing partial destruction of the septum pellucidum and damage to the hypothalamus. Endocrine abnormalities and schizencephaly are typical in this type of septo-optic dysplasia (see

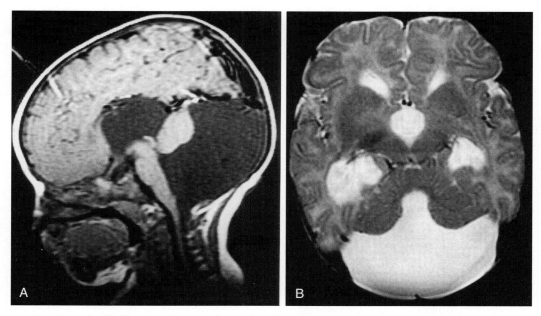

Figure 9–6. Dandy-Walker malformation. (*A* and *B*) MRI of a 6-month-old child with hydrocephalus. Both sagittal T1WI (*A*) and axial T2WI (*B*) show a large posterior fossa cyst that is continuous with the fourth ventricle. Enlarged third and lateral ventricles are visible on axial image (*B*). The sagittal image (*A*) also shows agenesis of the corpus callosum, which is occasionally associated with Dandy-Walker malformation. The entire posterior fossa is enlarged, with higher than normal location of the torcular (confluence of sinuses) and straight sinus.

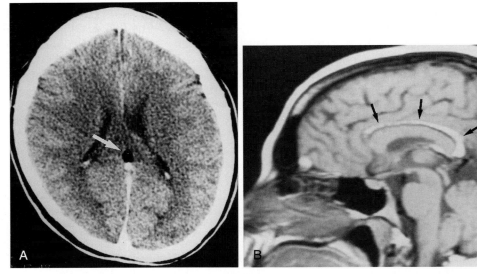

Figure 9–7. Lipoma of the corpus callosum. *(A)* On nonenhanced CT the lipoma is a rounded, low-density lesion just posterior to the corpus callosum *(arrow)*. *(B)* On sagittal T1-weighted MRI, the high signal intensity lipoma surrounds the corpus callosum *(arrows)*. Attenuation and signal characteristics are typical of fat.

Neuronal Migration Disorders, regarding schizencephaly). Coronal images demonstrate a box-like configuration of the frontal horns in septo-optic dysplasia, absence of the septum pellucidum, and, occasionally, identifiable hypoplasia of the optic nerves (Fig. 9–9).

Dandy-Walker and Other Cystic Malformations

Posterior fossa cystic malformations constitute a spectrum of disorders. Abnormal development of the fourth ventricle and/or cerebellum may result in the Dandy-Walker

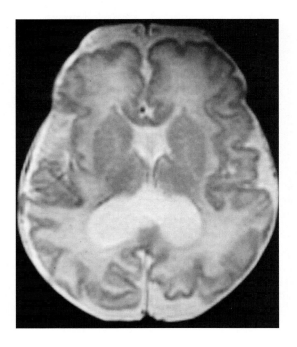

Figure 9–8. Holoprosencephaly. Axial MRI (T2WI) of a newborn with a mild (lobar) form of holoprosencephaly. The frontal horns are small and dysplastic, and there is no septum pellucidum.

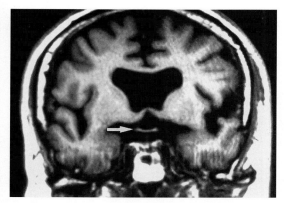

Figure 9–9. Septo-optic dysplasia. Coronal T1WI shows no septum pellucidum, box-like frontal horns, and small optic chiasm *(arrow).*

malformation, Dandy-Walker variant, or mega cisterna magna. The classic Dandy-Walker malformation includes a high tentorial attachment (above the lambdoid suture, also known as *torcular-lambdoid inversion*), severe or complete absence of the cerebellar vermis, and a large fourth ventricle opening into or constituting a large posterior fossa cyst (see Fig. 9–6). Hydrocephalus is common and accounts for many of the symptoms that occur. In the Dandy-Walker variant, less cerebellar hypoplasia occurs,

and the tentorium is not elevated. The fourth ventricle, however, is enlarged (Fig. 9–10). A mega cisterna magna, as the name implies, is manifested by an enlarged cisterna magna, with a normal fourth ventricle (Fig. 9–11). Patients with the Dandy-Walker variant and mega cisterna magna are much less likely to be symptomatic than those with Dandy-Walker malformation.

A midline retrocerebellar arachnoid cyst may be very difficult to distinguish from a mega cisterna magna without injection of contrast material into the subarachnoid space (a cisternogram). Arachnoid cysts may also occur elsewhere around the brain, with the anterior temporal region being a particularly common location (Fig. 9–12). Choroidal fissure cysts are benign cysts with a typical location and appearance (Fig. 9–13).

Neuronal Migration Disorders

Various injuries and errors of development can damage the central nervous system

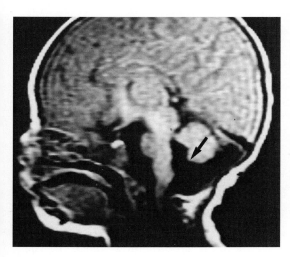

Figure 9–10. Dandy-Walker variant. MRI of a 1-month-old infant (sagittal T1WI). The fourth ventricle opens freely into a posterior fossa cyst *(arrow).* The straight sinus and torcular are normal in position.

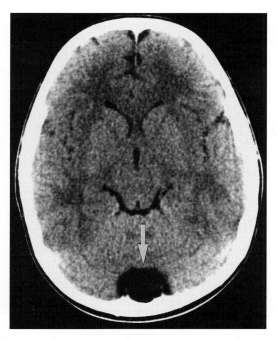

Figure 9–11. Mega cisterna magna. CT scan shows low density (CSF) in a large cisterna magna *(arrow).* The fourth ventricle is normal in size (not visible on this slice). A retrocerebellar arachnoid cyst may have a similar appearance.

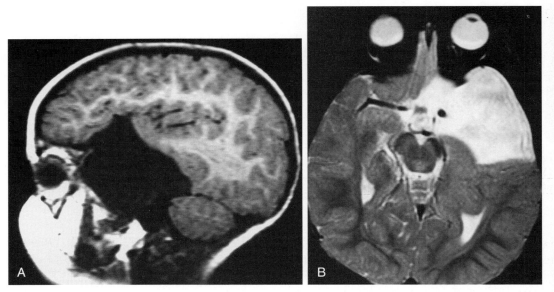

Figure 9–12. Arachnoid cyst. MRI of a child with an unusually large left temporal arachnoid cyst. *(A)* Sagittal T1WI through the left temporal lobe shows a dark fluid collection. *(B)* On axial T2WI, the fluid is bright. The cortex adjacent to the cyst is intact although displaced.

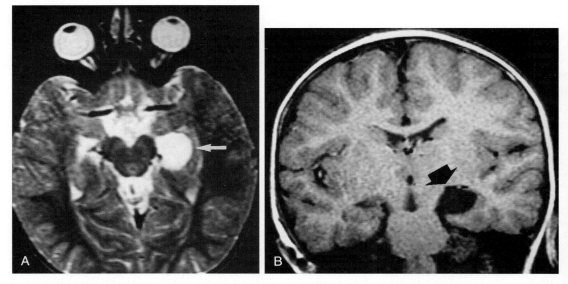

Figure 9–13. Choroidal fissure cyst. *(A)* MRI (axial T2WI) through the level of the temporal horns shows a rounded area of high signal intensity *(arrow)* adjacent to the left cerebral peduncle. *(B)* The coronal T1WI clarifies location within the left choroidal fissure *(arrow)*.

(CNS) during the period of neuroblast migration from the deep periventricular region to the cortex. Several types of migration abnormalities are recognized.

Heterotopia are focal or band-like rests of gray matter in abnormal locations deep to the cortex. On CT and MRI, they have identical attenuation or signal intensity compared with normal gray matter in the cortex (Fig. 9–14). The location of the gray matter rests is abnormal without evidence of associated edema or gliosis.

The term *schizencephaly* describes a complete cleft extending from ventricle to cortex and lined by gray matter. Clefts may be bilateral or unilateral and are further characterized as open-lip (Fig. 9–15) or closed-lip (Fig. 9–16), based on whether CSF is visible in the cleft or the sides of the cleft appear apposed. A dimple in the wall of a lateral ventricle may be a sign of a subtle closed-lip schizencephaly (see Fig. 9–16).

Agyria, pachygyria, and *lissencephaly* are all terms describing an abnormally smooth, thick cortex resulting from incomplete migration of the full neuronal layers of the cortex (Fig. 9–17). The condition may be widespread and bilateral or may be focal. Polymicrogyria, although characterized histologically by small gyri, often appears as a smooth cortical surface on gross physical inspection as well as on CT and MRI and may be difficult to distinguish from pachygyria. However, white matter damage or gliosis, anomalous veins, or deep clefts often accompany polymicrogyria but are absent in pachygyria (Fig. 9–18).

Unilateral megalencephaly is an unusual type of migration anomaly in which a hemisphere or portion of a hemisphere and the ipsilateral ventricle are enlarged.

The most common clinical manifestations of neuronal migration abnormalities are seizures and developmental delay. Most neuronal migration abnormalities are best visualized by MRI.

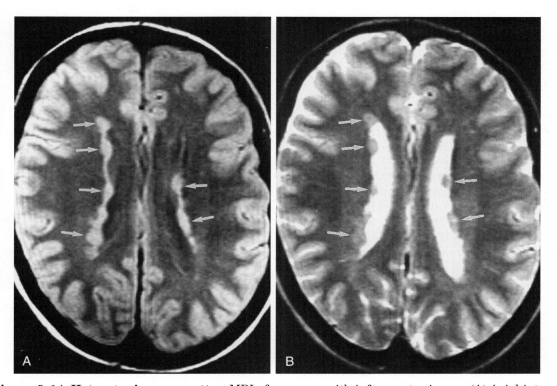

Figure 9–14. Heterotopic gray matter. MRI of a woman with infrequent seizures. *(A)* Axial intermediate view and *(B)* T2WI show multiple nodules *(arrows)* along the lateral margins of the lateral ventricles. The nodules have the same signal intensity as gray matter on all pulse sequences.

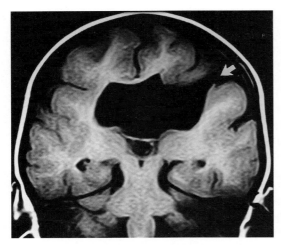

Figure 9–15. Open-lip schizencephaly. MRI (coronal T1WI) of a child shows CSF extending through an open cleft *(arrow)* in the left hemisphere. The septum pellucidum is absent.

NEUROCUTANEOUS SYNDROMES

Neurocutaneous syndromes may be considered a form of error in a later stage of CNS development—histogenesis. The most common neurocutaneous syndromes follow genetic patterns, often of autosomal dominant inheritance, and involve abnormalities of the CNS, skin, and often eyes. Other organ systems can be involved. The name *phakomatoses* is also applied to these conditions. (The term derives from the phakoma, a retinal lesion in tuberous sclerosis, but the term *phakomatosis* is less appropriate than *neurocutaneous syndrome,* in that phakomas seldom occur in syndromes other than tuberous sclerosis.) The most common and well-known of these diseases are neurofibromatosis, tuberous sclerosis, von Hippel-Lindau syndrome, and Sturge-Weber syndrome.

Neurofibromatosis

Neurofibromatosis is one of the most well-described and common human genetic syndromes. Because of the great variety in its clinical manifestations, it has only recently been shown that neurofibromatosis is comprised of more than one distinct entity. Al-though various subtypes have been described or proposed, two primary types are recognized, for which clinical diagnostic criteria and genetic characteristics have been defined (Tables 9–1, 9–2).

Neurofibromatosis type-1 (NF-1) is classic von Recklinghausen disease. It has an autosomal dominant pattern of transmission and results from a mutation on chromosome 17, with an incidence of approximately one in 3000 births. Clinical manifestations include CNS and visual symptoms, scoliosis and limb deformities, and the classic skin lesions of neurofibromas and café au lait spots. Ocular changes include the Lisch nodule, which is a pigmented hamartoma of the iris.

Several different abnormalities of the CNS occur with NF-1. Optic nerve gliomas and other gliomas of the visual tracts are particularly common and are usually but not always low-grade lesions. MRI is espe-

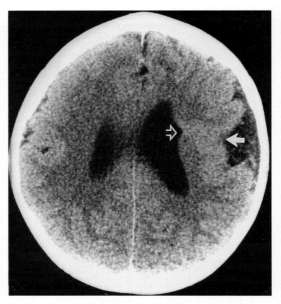

Figure 9–16. Closed-lip schizencephaly. Nonenhanced CT of a 4-year-old child with recent onset of seizure disorder. There is a contour change (dimple) in the lateral margin of the body of the left lateral ventricle *(open arrow).* Although the cleft is not directly visualized, there is gray matter extending from the ventricle to the surface of the brain *(between open and solid arrows).*

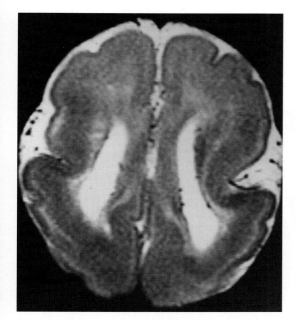

Figure 9–17. Pachygyria. MRI (axial T2WI) of a 6-month-old child with developmental delay and seizures. There are only a few shallow sulci present.

cially sensitive for detection of these gliomas (Fig. 9–19A). Astrocytomas of the CNS are also more common in patients with NF-1 than in the general population. MRI using gadolinium administration is the test of choice for evaluation of such tumors (see Fig. 4–3). Hydrocephalus may occur from obstruction of the cerebral aqueduct by tectal gliomas. The most common CNS imaging findings in NF-1 are small areas of high signal intensity on T2-weighted MR images in the brainstem, cerebellum, basal ganglia, and thalamus (Fig. 9–19B). The bright foci may be the result of delayed or abnormal myelination or hamartomas; they do not demonstrate contrast enhancement. Careful evaluation and sometimes follow-up imaging are necessary to distinguish these areas of increased signal from the edema accompanying a tumor. Plexiform neurofibromas may occur throughout the body, including the orbit and elsewhere in the skull, and present as infiltrative lesions that may deform bone.

Neurofibromas of the spine are common in NF-1, often appearing as dumbbell-shaped lesions enlarging a neural foramen and extending into the spinal canal (see Fig. 12–20). Lateral meningoceles are also common and may enlarge a neural foramen, as observed on plain film evaluation. CT or MRI readily distinguishes the fluid contents of a meningocele from a solid neoplasm. Kyphoscoliosis may occur spontaneously, often cervical or thoracic in location (Fig. 9–20), or may be related to a spinal tumor.

Neurofibromatosis-2 (NF-2) is only about one-tenth as common as NF-1. This autosomal dominant condition results from a mutation on chromosome 22. Skin lesions are

---

TABLE 9–1. Diagnostic Criteria for Neurofibromatosis-1*

The diagnosis of NF-1 may be made when *two or more* of the following are present:
1. Six or more cafe au lait macules whose greatest diameter is more than 5 mm in prepubertal patients and more than 15 mm in postpubertal patients
2. Two or more neurofibromas of any type or one plexiform neurofibroma
3. Freckling in the axillary or inguinal regions
4. Optic glioma
5. Two or more Lisch nodules (iris hamartomas)
6. A distinctive osseous lesion, such as sphenoid dysplasia or thinning of long-bone cortex
7. A parent, sibling, or child with neurofibromatosis-1 according to the criteria above

*Criteria established by a 1988 NIH Consensus Development Conference

---

TABLE 9–2. Diagnostic Criteria for Neurofibromatosis-2*

The diagnosis of NF-2 may be made when *one* of the following is present:
1. Bilateral eighth cranial nerve masses on CT or MRI
2. A parent, sibling, or child with NF-2 and either a unilateral eight cranial nerve mass or any two of the following: neurofibroma, meningioma, glioma, schwannoma, or juvenile posterior subcapsular lenticular opacity

*Criteria established by a 1988 NIH Consensus Development Conference

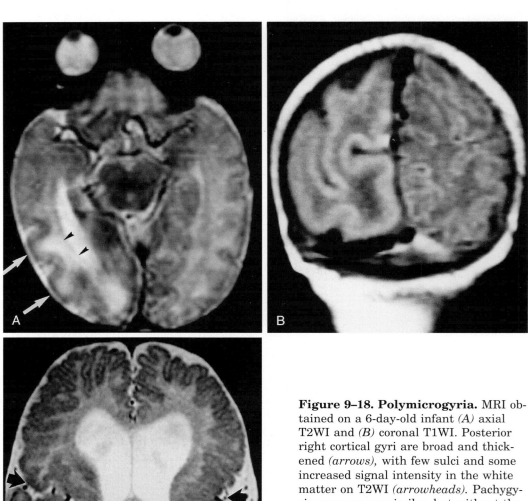

Figure 9–18. Polymicrogyria. MRI obtained on a 6-day-old infant *(A)* axial T2WI and *(B)* coronal T1WI. Posterior right cortical gyri are broad and thickened *(arrows),* with few sulci and some increased signal intensity in the white matter on T2WI *(arrowheads).* Pachygyria may appear similar, but without the white matter gliosis. *(C)* Axial T2WI of a 4-year-old child shows extensive polymicrogyria, with bilateral infolded cortical dysplasia manifested by deep clefts *(arrows).*

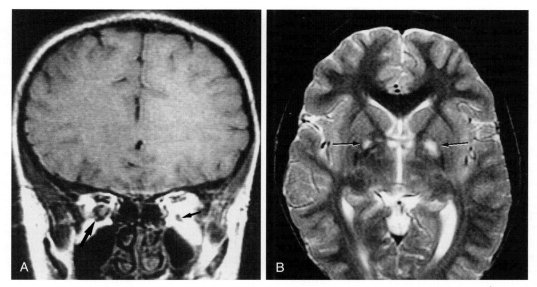

Figure 9–19. Neurofibromatosis-1, basal ganglia lesions and optic glioma. MRI of 9-year-old boy with NF-1. *(A)* Coronal T1WI shows enlarged right optic nerve *(large arrow)* resulting from an optic glioma. This is compared with the normal left optic nerve *(small arrow)*. *(B)* Axial T2WI of the same child shows bilateral, asymmetric bright areas in the globus pallidi *(arrows)*. These bright foci are very common in NF-1 and may also occur in the thalami, brainstem, and cerebellum.

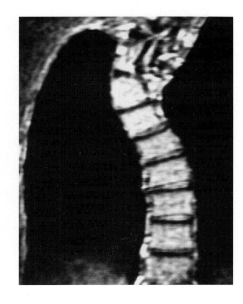

Figure 9–20. Scoliosis in neurofibromatosis-1. MRI (coronal T1WI) shows high thoracic scoliosis in a 37-year-old man with neurofibromatosis-1.

much less prominent than in NF-1. CNS manifestations are primarily cranial nerve schwannomas and meningiomas (Fig. 9–21). Eighth nerve schwannomas (acoustic neuromas) are common, and bilateral acoustic schwannomas in a young person are pathognomonic of NF-2 (see Table 9–2). Meningiomas are often multiple and may be intraventricular. In the spine, ependymomas of the spinal cord and neural sheath tumors are common and may be multiple. Contrast-enhanced MRI is the most sensitive imaging test for detection of nearly all of these tumors, most of which show some contrast enhancement (Fig. 9–22). A combination of sagittal and axial MRI best demonstrates the location (i.e., intramedullary or extramedullary/intradural) of a spinal tumor.

Tuberous Sclerosis

Tuberous sclerosis is inherited in an autosomal dominant pattern. The skin lesions of tuberous sclerosis are angiofibromas, commonly presenting on the cheeks (adenoma sebaceum), and ash-leaf macules. The phakoma is a common retinal lesion. Hamarto-

mas of the brain often result in seizures and developmental delay. The classic triad of adenoma sebaceum, seizures, and mental retardation is present in only about one-half of tuberous sclerosis patients. Cerebral hamartomas may occur in the cortex and subcortical white matter, and in the periventricular region. On MRI, these lesions are often observed as areas of altered signal intensity (Fig. 9–23), whereas on CT, calcification in cortical and periventricular lesions is a common observation (Fig. 9–24). Cortical lesions (tubers) cause widened gyri, and periventricular lesions alter the normally smooth contour of the ventricles. An unusual tumor, the subependymal giant cell astrocytoma, is specific to tuberous sclerosis. Because of its characteristic location near the foramen of Monro, this tumor often causes ventricular obstruction and consequent morbidity despite a low potential for malignant transformation (Fig. 9–25). Hamartomatous conditions of the kidneys (angiomyolipoma), heart (rhabdomyoma), and the lungs (lymphangiomyoma) may also occur. (Note that the lesions of tuberous sclerosis are essentially all hamartomas.)

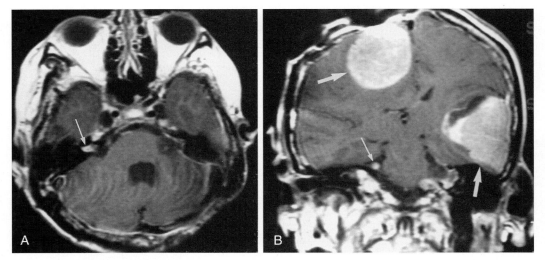

Figure 9–21. Neurofibromatosis-2, cranial findings. *(A)* MRI (post-gadolinium axial T1WI) shows enhancement of a recurrent acoustic schwannoma *(arrow)* in the right internal auditory canal (IAC). *(B)* Coronal T1WI of the same woman with NF-2 shows two large, enhancing meningiomas *(large arrows),* as well as a contrast-enhancing trigeminal schwannoma *(small arrow).* There has been prior surgery involving the left IAC. An enhancing mass adjacent to the left side of the pons is either another meningioma or a schwannoma of a lower cranial nerve.

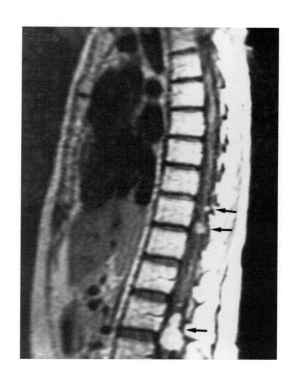

Figure 9–22. Neurofibromatosis-2, spinal tumors. MRI (post-gadolinium sagittal T1WI) of the thoracic spine demonstrates multiple enhancing masses *(arrows)* consistent with nerve sheath tumors. In addition, the patient had had a cervical intramedullary ependymoma resected in the past. There is an increased frequency of both nerve sheath tumors and ependymomas in NF-2.

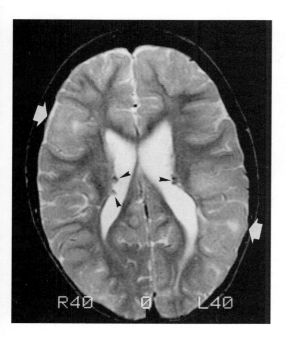

Figure 9–23. MR of tuberous sclerosis. Axial T2WI shows subependymal nodules *(arrowheads),* small white matter lesions, and cortical tubers. The latter are broad gyri with central increased signal intensity *(broad arrows).*

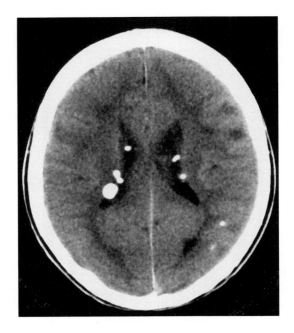

Figure 9–24. CT of tuberous sclerosis. Nonenhanced CT shows multiple calcifications of varying sizes in the periventricular white matter, as well as two left posterior cortical calcifications.

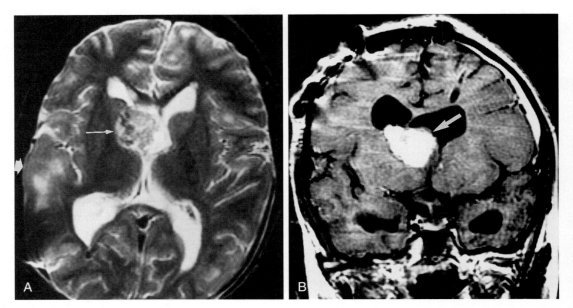

Figure 9–25. Subependymal giant-cell astrocytoma in tuberous sclerosis. MRI of 12-year-old girl with seizures, developmental delay, and worsening headaches. *(A)* Axial T2WI reveals a heterogeneous mass *(thin arrow)* adjacent to the foramen of Monro. (The superficial, right posterior low signal next to focus of bright signal is the result of metal artifact from previous surgery.) Broad gyrus with central high signal intensity *(broad arrow)* is a cortical tuber. *(B)* On coronal post-gadolinium T1WI, there is intense contrast enhancement of the tumor *(arrow)*. Bodies and temporal horns of the lateral ventricles are dilated because of obstruction by the tumor.

von Hippel-Lindau Syndrome

The von Hippel-Lindau syndrome, which is linked to chromosome 3, is characterized by retinal hemangiomas and hemangioblastomas of the CNS. The latter occur predominantly in the cerebellum, with spinal cord lesions less commonly observed. Hemangioblastomas elsewhere in the brain are rare. Hemangioblastomas are not unique to von Hippel-Lindau syndrome. Multiple hemangioblastomas, however, are among the diagnostic criteria that define this neurocutaneous syndrome.

Because the tumors of von Hippel-Lindau syndrome are highly vascular, they enhance intensely on both CT and MRI. They contain cystic elements in about two-thirds of cases. The cyst walls rarely enhance and do not contain neoplastic elements. The hemangioblastoma may present as an enhancing mural nodule along the margin of a cyst (see Fig. 4–11). A dense, prolonged stain is usually seen on angiography. Brain and spine tumors are responsible for neurologic changes based on their location. Because of a significant risk of renal cell carcinoma (a major cause of mortality in these patients), renal imaging should also be performed. Pheochromocytoma is also associated with von Hippel-Lindau syndrome, although at a lower incidence rate than renal cell carcinoma. Visceral cysts commonly occur in organs including the liver, spleen, adrenal glands, epididymis, and mesentery.

Sturge-Weber Syndrome

Sturge-Weber syndrome, unlike the previously described neurocutaneous syndromes, usually occurs sporadically, although various genetic patterns have also been described. Also known as *encephalotrigeminal angiomatosis,* this condition is defined by the combination of facial port-wine nevus and a leptomeningeal vascular malformation. These locations are related because of early developmental vascular anomalies involving the primitive brain and adjacent face. Glaucoma and congenital enlargement of the globe may result from involvement of the eye by the facial nevus. Impaired venous drainage of the brain leads to cortical atrophy and gyral tram-track calcifications. Seizures and developmental delay are common. CT and skull films demonstrate the typical calcifications (Fig. 9–26), and contrast-enhanced MRI reveals gyral-type enhancement in the same distribution.

PERINATAL PROBLEMS

Intracranial hemorrhage and periventricular leukomalacia, two common problems in premature infants, are initially best evaluated with sonography. Cranial ultrasound testing has several advantages in the infant. The open fontanelle provides an acoustic window. The examination may be performed at the bedside in the intensive care unit without sedation, and the cost is less than that of CT or MRI. Serial follow-up of complications such as hydrocephalus is facilitated (Fig. 9–27). CT and MRI are usually reserved for complicated or ambiguous cases and for later follow-up if necessary.

The continuing successes of neonatal intensive care medicine have resulted in increasing numbers of infants surviving premature birth. The immature brain is susceptible to unique problems. The germinal matrix, which lies near the ventricular system, is present until the end of the second trimester, when it begins involution. Hemorrhages are common in this region. Germinal matrix hemorrhage is generally graded using four levels of severity (Table 9–3), depending on whether there is ventricular or parenchymal hemorrhage and

TABLE 9–3. Grading of Germinal Matrix Hemorrhage in Premature Infants

Grade I	Germinal matrix hemorrhage (subependymal)
Grade II	Intraventricular hemorrhage, normal-size ventricles
Grade III	Intraventricular hemorrhage, enlarged ventricles
Grade IV	Parenchymal hemorrhage involving cerebral hemispheres

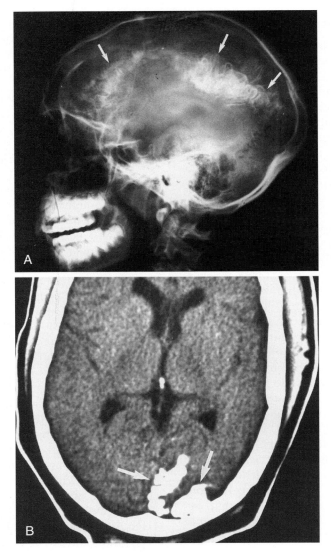

Figure 9–26. Calcifications in Sturge-Weber syndrome. *(A)* Lateral plain film of a patient with Sturge-Weber syndrome shows gyriform, "tram-track" calcifications *(arrows)*. *(B)* Axial nonenhanced CT of a different patient demonstrates similar calcification in the left occipital lobe *(arrows)*.

whether or not the ventricles are dilated. Risk of long-term neurologic damage increases with higher grades of hemorrhage. Initial screening sonography is often performed in premature infants, with additional scans as needed (Fig. 9–28). Hemorrhage is visualized as a region of increased echogenicity (hyperechoic), which is typically near the caudothalamic groove (near the caudate head). Normal choroid plexus is also echogenic but lies posterior to the caudothalamic groove. Ventricular and parenchymal hemorrhage and hydrocephalus can also be identified with and followed by sonography.

A second common injury to the brain in premature infants is periventricular leukomalacia. Clinically, this is often associated with various forms of cerebral palsy. The combination of immature vascularity, with different boundary or watershed zones as compared with the mature pattern, and

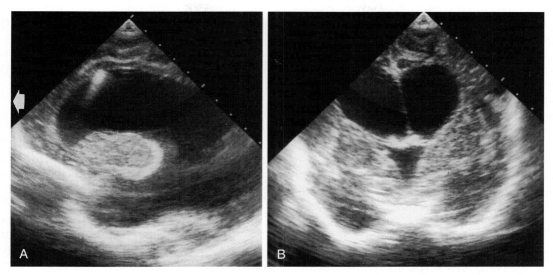

Figure 9–27. Ultrasound study of hydrocephalus. Cranial ultrasound of a newborn infant. Marked dilatation of the lateral ventricles is visible on *(A)* parasagittal and *(B)* coronal views, with the third ventricle also visible on the latter. The arrow in *A* points anteriorly.

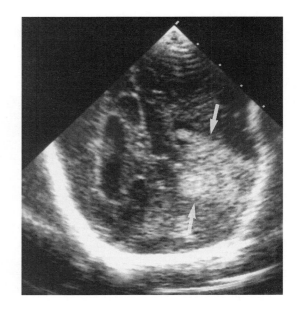

Figure 9–28. Intraventricular and parenchymal hemorrhage in a premature infant. Coronal ultrasound of a premature infant who had a germinal matrix hemorrhage (grade IV). Hemorrhage in the left lateral ventricle and adjacent parenchyma *(arrows)* appears echogenic (bright).

hypoxia make the periventricular region susceptible to ischemia in premature infants. Infarction in the deep white matter, which is typically near the frontal horns and atria of the lateral ventricles, results in edema, frequent hemorrhage, and, ultimately, cavitation and cyst formation. Hyperechoic areas are present with edema (Fig. 9–29A). Follow-up in several weeks demonstrates cystic changes (Fig. 9–29B). Late changes on CT or MRI include focal areas of volume loss, ventricular enlargement, and irregularity of the margins of the lateral ventricles.

Arterial infarction in the perinatal period can result in encephalomalacia in vascular territories. These infarctions are readily observed on CT and MRI.

POSTNATAL ACQUIRED DISORDERS OF THE BRAIN

Trauma

Cranial trauma is discussed in Chapter 2. The imaging abnormalities are generally similar for children and adults. Child abuse, however, deserves special attention. Over 2000 children are estimated to die of abuse and neglect in the United States each year. Although there is increased risk of child abuse in groups under greater conditions of stress, no racial or socioeconomic group is exempt.

Any evidence of significant injury to a child without adequate explanation must raise the possibility of nonaccidental trauma.

Trivial head injuries are common in infants and toddlers, but significant intracranial injury rarely results from minor falls in otherwise healthy children. Mechanisms of brain injury in child abuse include direct blows and shaking or whiplash injury. Hence, the terms *battered child* and *shaken baby syndrome* are often applied. Strangulation can also be a factor. Retinal hemorrhages are an important clinical sign of a shaking injury. Multiple, complex, or depressed skull fractures (Fig. 9–30), bilateral or interhemispheric subdural hematomas (Figs. 9–30, 9–31), and contusions in a child without a clear history of major trauma strongly suggest the diagnosis of child abuse. As with injuries elsewhere in the body, multiple intracranial injuries or injuries of varying ages provide evidence of repeated trauma.

Both noncontrasted CT and MRI can be helpful and are complementary in cases of suspected child abuse. CT is more sensitive than MRI for subarachnoid hemorrhage and is excellent for acute parenchymal hemorrhage as well. MRI is more sensitive for

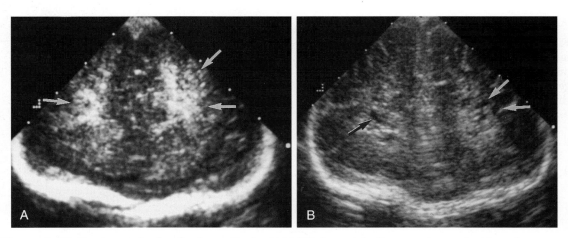

Figure 9–29. Periventricular leukomalacia. *(A)* Initial cranial ultrasound examination of a premature infant, coronal plane through the frontal lobes, shows echogenic (bright) edema *(arrows)* near the frontal horns. *(B)* Follow-up examination 3 weeks later, also in the coronal plane, reveals interval development of small cysts (leukomalacia, *arrows*). (Courtesy of Dr. J. Biernacki.)

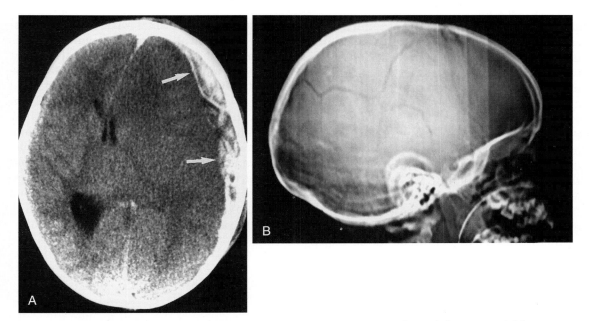

Figure 9–30. Child abuse. *(A)* CT scan of a 2-year-old child shows a large left extra-axial hematoma with mixed attenuation *(arrows),* edema of the left cerebral hemisphere, interhemispheric blood, and severe shift of the midline to the right. *(B)* Localizing digital CT scout image shows a large, stellate skull fracture.

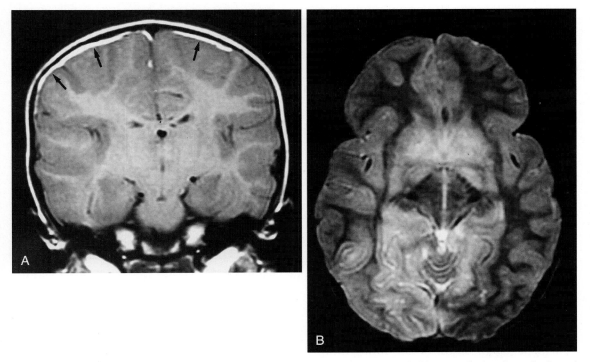

Figure 9–31. Child abuse. MRI obtained 5 days after this 3-year-old child was admitted to the hospital with head and abdominal injuries. *(A)* On coronal T1WI, thin bilateral and interhemispheric subdural hematomas are visible as bright layers over both cerebral convexities *(arrows)* and in the interhemispheric fissure. *(B)* Axial T2WI shows subtle increased signal intensity in the basal ganglia and thalami and in the occipital and posterior temporal cortex from ischemia. History included blows to the head.

shearing injury, small contusions, and small subdural hematomas. MRI can be especially useful in establishing the presence of hematomas of differing ages, either extra-axial or intra-axial types. Cerebral ischemia can also result from child abuse and can be demonstrated with either CT or MRI (see Fig. 9–31). Skull films may be necessary for diagnosing skull fractures. As previously noted in Chapter 2, skull films are not obtained for evaluation of the brain; CT and MRI are used for this purpose. Rather, skull fractures are sought because they serve as evidence of physical injury. For this reason, skull films are often obtained as part of a complete skeletal survey in cases of suspected child abuse.

Many states have mandatory reporting requirements to protective service agencies if child abuse is suspected.

Other Acquired Conditions

Intracranial infections are discussed in Chapter 3. Important perinatal infections are from toxoplasmosis, cytomegalovirus, herpes, and human immunodeficiency virus.

Intracranial neoplasms are discussed in Chapter 4. Posterior fossa tumors are common in childhood, and the differential diagnosis of posterior fossa masses, especially those causing obstruction of the ventricular system at the level of the fourth ventricle, is discussed in Chapter 7. Neoplasms that are congenital or that appear very early in life are uncommon, and the differential diagnosis differs from that in older age groups. Teratomas, primitive neuroectodermal tumors (PNET), choroid plexus papillomas, medulloblastomas, and hypothalamic astrocytomas should be considered.

Degenerative diseases of childhood are rare, but they sometimes have a distinctive imaging appearance. A brief overview is presented in Chapter 8.

Mesial temporal sclerosis is a condition in which degeneration of the hippocampus leads to temporal lobe seizures. The etiology is uncertain but may be the result of ischemia or other insult in childhood. Seizures may begin early or as late as adulthood. Because surgical resection is occasionally

considered for patients with seizures resistant to medical therapy, imaging is important. Along with electroencephalography, MRI can aid in localizing the site of abnormality. High resolution imaging is helpful (Fig. 9–32). Coronal or oblique coronal images through the temporal lobe may show the affected hippocampus to be smaller than normal. Loss of definition of internal structure and abnormally increased signal intensity are occasionally observed. Apparent enlargement of the medial temporal lobe or a more extensive area of signal abnormality should raise the suspicion of astrocytoma.

CRANIOSYNOSTOSIS

Major sutures of the skull include the sagittal, coronal, lambdoid, and metopic sutures. Premature closure of one or more sutures

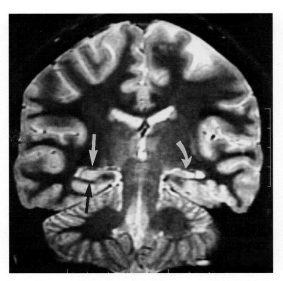

Figure 9–32. Mesial temporal (hippocampal) sclerosis. MRI of a 25-year-old woman with temporal lobe seizures following childhood meningitis. T2WI perpendicular (oblique coronal) to the long axis of the temporal lobes shows normal anatomy of the right hippocampus *(between straight arrows),* an oval gray-matter structure in the medial temporal lobe, just below the choroidal fissure. The hippocampus on the patient's left side *(curved arrow)* is small and indistinct, with a region of increased signal intensity.

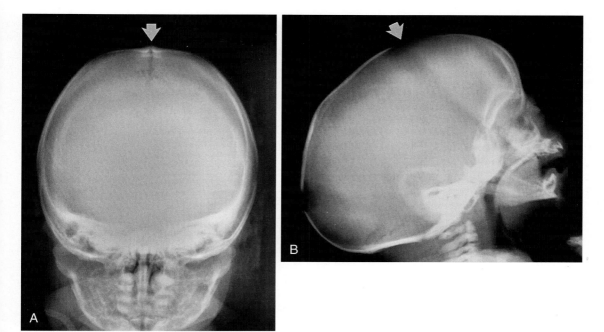

Figure 9–33. Craniosynostosis. AP *(A)* and lateral skull radiographs *(B)* of a child with sagittal synostosis show bone bridging *(A)* the sagittal suture *(arrow)* and a disproportionately long skull (scaphocephaly or dolichocephaly) *(B)*. The coronal suture remains widely open *(B, arrow)*.

results in deformity of the skull. Growth along the fused suture stops, and increased growth takes place along other sutures. Sagittal synostosis is most common and results in an elongated skull (dolichocephaly, scaphocephaly). The coronal suture is next most commonly involved. Coronal synostosis results in a shortened skull (brachycephaly). Unilateral or asymmetric synostosis of the coronal or lambdoid sutures can occur, resulting in asymmetry of the head. The diagnosis can often be made on the basis of clinical examination. Skull radiographs are usually adequate to confirm the skull deformity and asymmetry of the sutures (Fig. 9–33). CT is helpful in some cases, especially for lambdoid synostosis, and occasionally is used for surgical planning. In addition to isolated synostosis occurring as a developmental error, multiple synostoses can accompany genetic syndromes. CT or MRI of the brain may be indicated to evaluate associated abnormalities such as ventriculomegaly.

10

Approach to Imaging the Spine: Anatomy, Development, and Disorders of Development

The spinal cord is subject to many of the same diseases as the brain. However, considerable differences occur in frequency of these conditions because of anatomic and pathophysiologic variations. Unlike the brain, intrinsic disease of the spinal cord is relatively uncommon, whereas nearby processes that impinge upon the spinal cord, nerve roots, or spinal nerves occur frequently. Because degenerative conditions and trauma are common, mechanical injuries related to the vertebral column in particular are very important in spinal cord disease. The focus of this book is on neurologic rather than musculoskeletal disease. However, some consideration must be given to diseases of the spine itself. An approach to imaging of the spine and congenital disorders is presented in this chapter. Traumatic injuries of the spine are discussed in Chapter 11. Other acquired nontraumatic disorders of the spine are examined in Chapter 12.

APPROACH TO SPINAL IMAGING

Anatomy

Because of the importance of both osseous and neural elements in the spine, plain films, CT, and MRI all have appropriate uses. Normal plain-film anatomy of the cervical spine is illustrated in Chapter 11. Normal sagittal MRI of the cervical spine demonstrates the marrow space, the intervertebral discs, and spinal cord (Fig. 10–1).

Blood is supplied to the spinal cord by a midline anterior artery and two posterolateral arteries. In the thoracic and lumbar regions, a radiculomedullary branch (the artery of Adamkiewicz) provides the primary arterial supply to the anterior spinal cord. In about 75 percent of patients, this artery arises from the left side between T9 and T12. Locating the level and side of this artery is important in some cases, especially for surgical planning. The artery has a characteristic hairpin configuration (Fig. 10–2).

Classification by Compartments

Before discussing individual diseases, it is useful to consider the approach to imaging spine disease and radiographic classification of such diseases. A broad separation, based on compartments, is very useful. These compartments are (1) intramedullary (within the spinal cord); (2) extramedullary intradural (outside the spinal cord but within the thecal sac); and (3) extradural (outside the dura mater) (Fig. 10–3). Earlier

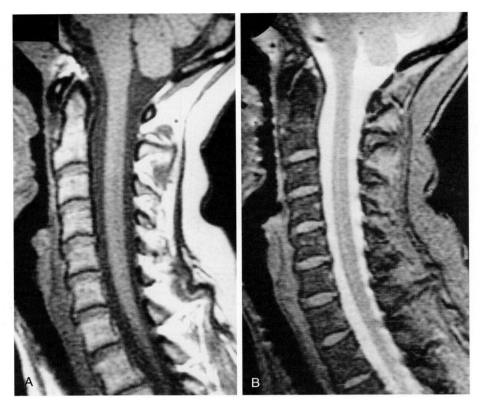

Figure 10–1. Normal MRI cervical spine. Midline sagittal T1WI *(A)* and T2WI *(B)*.

radiographic criteria emphasized factors observed on myelography. Myelography, however, is currently used much less frequently than in the past. Categorizing lesions according to these three compartments remains very useful because the differential diagnosis is distinct for each.

Intramedullary Processes

Intramedullary processes are best visualized with MRI. Abnormalities include (1) altered contour of the spinal cord, either expanded or contracted; (2) altered signal intensity; and (3) contrast enhancement (under normal conditions, no enhancement of the spinal cord is observed).

Myelography is invasive but shows the spinal cord outlined by intrathecal contrast material. Intramedullary disease is recognized myelographically by alteration of the contour and size of the spinal cord. CT alone is very insensitive to spinal cord pathology, but CT following myelography shows the size and shape of the spinal cord well. In

addition, delayed CT following myelography can show contrast media entering syrinx cavities.

Common intramedullary processes are listed in Table 10–1. Neoplasms are the most common of this group, but syrinx, myelitis, and vascular disease are also important.

Extramedullary Intradural Processes

Extramedullary intradural diseases deviate or impinge upon the spinal cord without indenting the dura mater. Neurofibromas and meningiomas are the most common conditions of the group presented in Table 10–2. CT-myelography and MRI are both effective in demonstrating these conditions (Fig. 10–4). Neurofibromas in particular are often mixed in location, with extension into the adjacent neural foramen. "Drop" metastases of certain CNS neoplasms, which are spread via cerebrospinal fluid pathways, are also in this class.

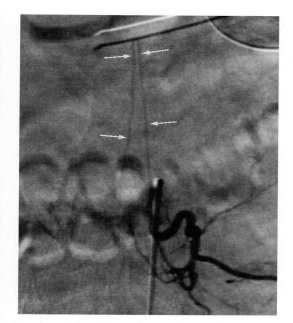

Figure 10–2. Normal anterior spinal artery. Preoperative AP digital subtraction angiogram of a left lower thoracic origin spinal artery. The artery has a typical hairpin configuration *(arrows).*

Extradural Processes

A large number of extradural processes can affect the spinal cord or nerves (Table 10–3). A herniated nucleus pulposus of an intervertebral disc is one of the most common. Others include metastasis, abscess, hematoma, and a variety of processes originating in the bone (see Chapter 12). Location outside the dura mater can be recognized via myelography, CT, or MRI.

CONGENITAL SPINE DISORDERS

Overview

Formation of the spine and its contents is conveniently considered as three processes: (1) neurulation, (2) canalization and retrogressive differentiation, and (3) formation of the vertebral column.

Neurulation includes formation of a neural plate, folding of that plate to form a neural tube, and separation (disjunction) of overlying ectoderm that forms skin. General categories of errors that can occur during this process include failure of the neural tube to close, premature disjunction, and focal failure of disjunction.

Canalization is a complex process responsible for formation of the conus medullaris and filum terminale. A caudal cell mass distal to the neural tube forms an ependymal-lined tube that unites with the neural tube, followed by retrogressive differentiation and cell necrosis. Insults or errors during this process affect the distal spinal cord or filum terminale.

A process of sclerotome formation, chondrification, and ossification leads to development of the vertebral column. Anomalies of the vertebral column are common as isolated occurrences but are also frequently associated with congenital spinal cord ab-

SPACES OF THE SPINAL CANAL

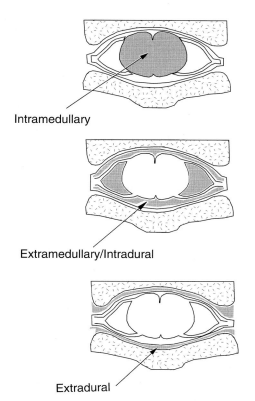

Intramedullary

Extramedullary/Intradural

Extradural

Figure 10–3. Spaces of the spinal canal. The three major compartments of the spinal canal are shown in the shaded area of each cross-sectional diagram.

TABLE 10–1. **Diseases of the Spine: Intramedullary Compartment**

Neoplasm
  Ependymoma—especially in conus medullaris
    and filum terminale
  Astrocytoma—mostly low-grade
  Hemangioblastoma—uncommon, highly vascular
Syrinx
  Syringomyelia (a fluid-filled cavity within the
    spinal cord, not lined by ependyma)
  Hydromyelia (a fluid-filled, enlarged central
    canal, lined by ependyma)
  The pathologic distinction between
    syringomyelia and hydromyelia is usually not
    distinguishable on imaging; the term "syrinx"
    or "syringohydromyelia" includes both (See
    Chapter 12)
Hematoma
Multiple sclerosis
Transverse myelitis

normalities. Split notochord syndromes in which the cord is divided (for example, in diastematomyelia) are rarely observed.

Open Neural Tube Defects

Open neural tube defects are nearly always clinically obvious. Myelomeningoceles of the spine occur in approximately 0.6 per 1000 births. The lumbar spine is the most common location by far, although cervical and thoracic myelomeningoceles can occur rarely. In open spinal dysraphism, there is

TABLE 10–2. **Diseases of the Spine: Intradural Extramedullary Compartment**

Neoplasms
  Nerve sheath tumors (neurofibroma and
    schwannoma)
  Meningioma
    (These two groups constitute over 80 to 90%
      of masses in this compartment)
  "Drop" metastases
  Dermoid and epidermoid
Lipoma
Arachnoid cysts
Foreign material (retained Pantopaque)

TABLE 10–3. **Diseases of the Spine: Extradural Compartment**

Herniated nucleus pulposus (most common)
Abscess
Hematoma
Vertebral metastasis
Other diseases originating in vertebrae
  Paget's disease
  Primary bone tumors

protrusion of spinal canal contents through a skin defect. The normal process of neurulation (through which the neural plate folds, forms a tube, and separates from overlying ectoderm) does not occur. Therefore, the end of the neural plate remains flattened and attached to the adjacent skin surface. The exposed neural tissue is termed a *neural placode*. Because of the lateral attachment to ectoderm that ultimately forms the skin, the usual ascent of the spinal cord relative to the spine cannot occur (Fig. 10–5). Despite early surgery, the termination of the spinal cord remains very low, and scarring may cause clinical symptoms of tethering later in life. Nerve roots extend from the ventral surface of the neural placode. Some neurologic impairment always exists, but the degree of severity is variable. The extent of neurologic impairment is related more to the level of spinal nerve involvement than to focal imaging or anatomic findings. Myelomeningocele is nearly always associated with the Chiari II malformation (see Chapter 9). Clinical aspects are therefore closely tied to coexisting hydrocephalus and shunt complications.

Postnatal imaging of the spine has a limited role in myelomeningocele. Initial diagnosis can often be made with prenatal ultrasound tests. A complete prenatal ultrasound examination includes evaluation of the entire spine for the presence of posterior elements. Focal widening of the pedicles is an important clue to the presence of spina bifida. Following delivery and after surgical covering of the defect, subsequent spine imaging is primarily directed toward complications, such as tethering of the spinal cord and scoliosis. MRI is particularly suitable

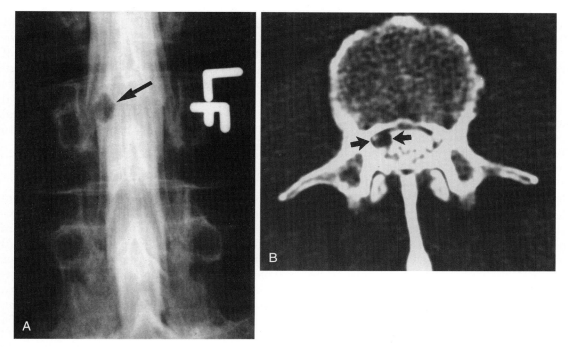

Figure 10–4. Nerve root tumor. Neural tumor is visible as an intradural filling defect *(arrows)* on a myelogram at the L4 level on the patient's right *(A)* and on a post-myelogram CT scan *(B)*.

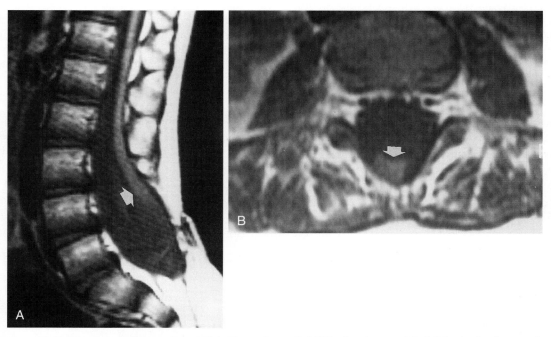

Figure 10–5. Myelomeningocele and tethered cord. MRI of a 6-year-old child who had a myelomeningocele repaired. *(A)* On the sagittal T1WI, the spinal cord *(arrow)* extends distally into an enlarged spinal canal. The posterior elements are absent in the distal lumbar spine. Nerve roots may simulate the appearance of the spinal cord on sagittal images, and another plane is important *(B, axial T1WI)* to confirm the findings *(arrow,* spinal cord at the L4 level).

for evaluation of the spinal cord (see Fig. 10–5).

Premature Disjunction

Despite some similarities, lipomyelomeningoceles differ in important ways from myelomeningoceles. Lipomyelomeningoceles are not associated with Chiari malformations. They originate later in gestation, following neural tube folding and separation of the tube from overlying ectoderm. Premature disjunction, before the neural tube has completely formed, results in the interior of the tube being exposed to mesenchyme. Developing nervous tissue that is exposed to mesenchyme in this manner is induced to form fat (lipoma). The spinal cord again terminates in a neural placode (attached to lipoma) and extends caudal to the usual termination at L2. There is, however, an intact covering of skin. Detection may occur much later in life. MRI and CT can both reveal the distal lipoma, occult spina bifida, and low-lying spinal cord, but MRI is better for evaluation of the spinal cord itself (Fig. 10–6). Symptoms such as lower extremity motor or sensory deficits or changes in bowel or bladder function are the result of tethering of the spinal cord.

Lipomas of the filum terminale are occasionally seen as incidental findings on MRI and are often clinically insignificant. However, there may be an increased incidence of tethered cord with such lipomas. Intradural lipomas are uncommon lesions, which are usually located in the thoracic or cervical spinal cord. They occur in an intradural subpial location. The lipoma lies adjacent to the dorsal surface of the spinal cord.

Failure of Disjunction

Focal failure of disjunction of ectoderm from the neural tube causes a dorsal dermal sinus. A canal or tube lined with epithelium extends from the skin toward the spinal cord. A defect is present in the posterior elements of the spine. Such sinuses can terminate in subcutaneous tissue, the dura mater, the subarachnoid space, a nerve root, or the spinal cord itself. Approximately 50 percent terminate in dermoid or epidermoid cysts; however, only 20 to 30 percent of epidermoid and dermoid cysts of the spine are related to dermal sinus tracts. These sinuses are a potential route of infection, which is a common reason for clinical presentation. A midline dimple in the skin is visible, often associated with a hyperpigmented patch, capillary angioma, or tuft of hair. These clinical findings are indications

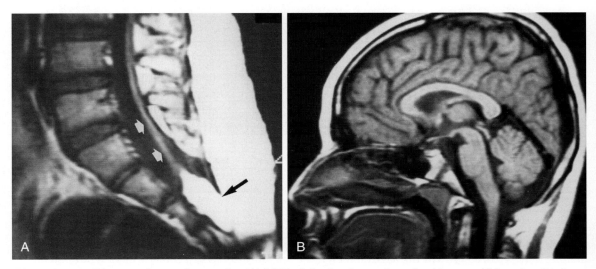

Figure 10–6. Lipomyelomeningocele. *(A)* MRI of the lumbar spine of a 10-year-old boy (sagittal T1WI) shows high signal intensity of fat in distal lipoma *(black arrow).* The spinal cord is tethered and extends into the sacral spinal canal *(white arrows).* *(B)* Sagittal MRI of the head (T1WI) is normal, with no Chiari malformation.

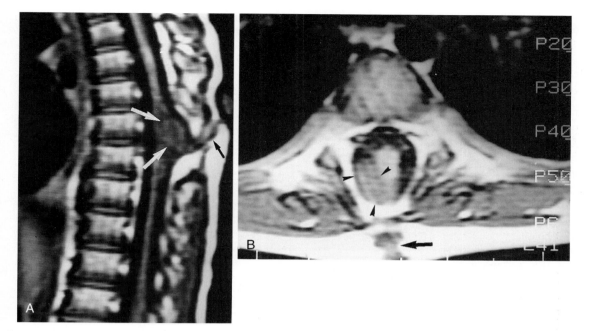

Figure 10–7. Dorsal dermal sinus, dermoid cyst. MRI of a 2-year-old who presented with a draining sinus on her back. *(A)* Sagittal T1WI shows a tract *(black arrow)* extending from the skin to a mass in the spinal canal *(white arrows)*. *(B)* Axial long TR/short TE image shows part of the sinus tract in the subcutaneous tissue *(arrow)*. An intermediate signal intensity mass *(arrowheads)* lying posterolateral to the spinal cord was found at surgery to be a dermoid cyst.

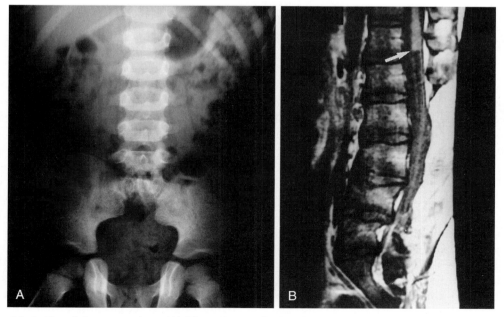

Figure 10–8. Caudal regression. *(A)* There is very little of the sacrum present on an AP radiograph at the age of 2 years. *(B)* MRI obtained 13 years later (sagittal T1WI) again shows a rudimentary small sacrum. There is abnormally high and abrupt termination of the conus medullaris *(arrow)* at T12.

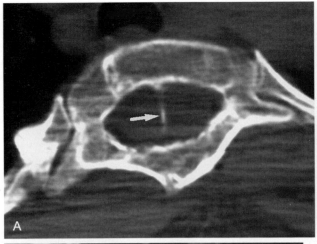

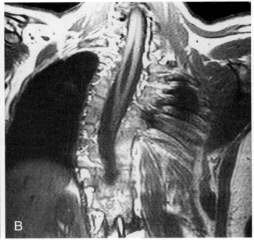

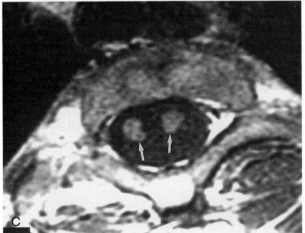

Figure 10–9. Diastematomyelia. *(A)* CT scan through the upper thoracic spine reveals an ossified septum *(arrow)* extending across the spinal canal. The vertebral body is abnormal, and there were multiple fused vertebral bodies. (*B* and *C*) Division into two hemicords *(arrows)* is clearly visible on T1-weighted MRI (coronal *(B)* and axial *(C)* images).

for imaging. MRI is the best test because of its multiplanar capability and superior soft tissue discrimination (Fig. 10–7). CT may also show a tract.

Abnormal Canalization

A tethered spinal cord can occur in association with various conditions, including myelomeningocele and lipomyelomeningocele. It can also occur as a result of abnormal development of the distal spine. Symptoms include bladder dysfunction, lower extremity weakness and abnormal reflexes, and back pain. Symptoms may appear at any age. The tip of the conus medullaris usually lies no lower than L2-L3 after 3 months of age and is usually above the mid-L2 level. Diagnosis is readily made noninvasively with MRI. Sagittal images, although they may

suggest the abnormality, are unreliable because the nerve roots of the cauda equina may be indistinguishable from the conus medullaris. Another plane of imaging is necessary, and T1-weighted axial images are usually helpful in identifying the end of the conus medullaris (see Fig. 10–5). A tight thickened filum terminale larger than 2 mm in diameter is often observed.

Other anomalies related to errors of canalization and retrogressive differentiation are caudal regression syndromes and teratomas. Caudal regression includes a spectrum ranging from mild abnormalities to complete sacral or even lumbar agenesis. Associated abnormalities of the genitourinary and gastrointestinal systems are common. There is an association with maternal diabetes, which accounts for about one case in six. Radiographs are helpful for the evaluation of the extent of bone abnormalities (Fig. 10–8A). MRI demonstrates an abnormally high termination of the spinal cord, often with an unusual wedge-like or squared-off configuration (Fig. 10–8B).

Sacrococcygeal teratomas are rare tumors arising from rests of cells in the caudal cell mass. They involve the lower sacrum and may be either external or internal (pelvic) masses. Approximately two-thirds are mature teratomas, with the others being immature or anaplastic. The mixture of internal tissues and materials, ranging from fat to calcium, results in a heterogeneous mass on cross-sectional imaging by either CT or MRI.

Split Notochord Syndromes

Diastematomyelia is the most common manifestation of the split notochord syndrome. Much rarer conditions include dorsal enteric fistula and enteric cyst, which is a rare intraspinal mass. Diastematomyelia refers to a sagittal division of the spinal cord into two hemicords. The two hemicords can lie either within a single dural sac, or the arachnoid and dura mater can also be split and create two separate sacs. In the latter case, a cartilaginous or bony spur commonly extends sagittally across the spinal canal. The spinal cord nearly always rejoins. Symptoms usually are related to tethering of the spinal cord. Clubfoot is present in about one half of symptomatic patients, and cutaneous stigmata commonly overlie the level of abnormality. Bony abnormalities are nearly always present, including spina bifida, fusion of lamina of adjacent vertebrae (termed *intersegmental laminar fusion*), vertebral body anomalies (such as hemivertebrae and butterfly vertebrae), and kyphoscoliosis.

Because of the complexity of diastematomyelia, more than one imaging technique may be necessary. Radiographs reveal the bony abnormalities, and CT may be necessary to see a bony spur through the canal (Fig. 10–9A). MRI is superior for visualizing the split spinal cord itself; multiple planes, such as coronal and axial, are advantageous (Fig. 10–9B,C). Although bony spurs may be observed with MRI, especially with gradient echo techniques, CT is much more reliable for identifying calcified structures.

Chapter

11

Spinal Trauma

Spine injuries are a major source of morbidity and mortality. Motor vehicle accidents contribute to a large share of such injuries, but there are many other causes. There are significant differences in the types of injuries occurring in various regions of the spine (see Table 11–1). It is also helpful to consider the directional forces most likely involved in producing spine injuries. The deduced mechanism of injury (flexion, extension, lateral bending, compression, or distraction) may be useful in both clinical and radiographic assessment. When a patient with trauma is suspected of having suffered a spine injury, both clinical evaluation and imaging are crucial.

Spine injuries are significant for both mechanical (structural) and neurologic implications. Structural integrity of the spine depends on adequate bony support and soft tissue support from ligaments, tendons, muscles, and intervertebral discs. Radiographs (plain films), CT, and MRI are complementary in the evaluation of spine trauma, and each has utility in specific situations. Radiographic studies (plain films and CT) are especially sensitive to the bony elements; MRI is especially sensitive to soft tissue injury of the discs, ligaments, and neural elements.

Plain films are excellent for depiction of many spine fractures and the alignment of the spine. They are also easily obtained and relatively inexpensive. Hence, plain films serve as the first imaging test in most trauma evaluations.

CT is more sensitive than plain films for fractures of the posterior elements. Details of bone displacement are visualized well with CT. If the patient stays immobile during imaging, reconstruction of two- and three-dimensional views can be performed. Limitations of CT are apparent with fractures that lie primarily parallel to the plane of imaging (the axial plane), such as odontoid and Chance fractures.

MRI has limited sensitivity for fractures but high sensitivity for soft tissue injury. It is the imaging study of choice for most spinal cord injuries, showing both spinal cord compression and intramedullary edema and hemorrhage. MRI may also yield very useful information regarding ligamentous injury, disc disruption, and vascular occlusion. Chronic spinal cord responses to injury, such as myelomalacia (atrophy) and syrinx formation (a fluid-filled cavity within the spinal cord), are best imaged with MRI (see Chapter 12 for a discussion of the differential diagnosis of syrinx). Obtaining MRI poses a greater technical challenge in trauma patients than does obtaining plain films or CT images.

Currently, myelography has a more limited use than in the past. It is primarily useful when MRI cannot be obtained or when specific problem-solving situations occur.

EVALUATION OF THE CERVICAL SPINE

Complete plain film evaluation of the cervical spine extends from the skull base to the upper thoracic spine. The C7-T1 junction and cervicocranial junction are potential pitfalls in imaging. The cervicothoracic junction is often difficult to visualize on a lateral view, and additional views, such as the swimmer's view or oblique views, can be very helpful (Fig. 11–1). A crosstable lateral view is often obtained initially, using portable technique when necessary. There is no consensus on which views to include in a routine trauma study, but usually lateral, anteroposterior (AP), and odontoid views are included in a complete study. Oblique or pillar views are occasionally obtained, espe-

cially for improved visualization of the posterior elements.

Lateral radiographs of the neck with patient-controlled flexion and extension can be employed. These serve as tests of ligamentous integrity. However, the limitations of these views (that involve patient movement) must be understood. There is risk to the patient if an unstable injury is present. Flexion-extension views obtained immediately after injury are often nondiagnostic because of muscle spasm or involuntary guarding that limits motion. Motion studies are more reliable several weeks after an injury. Immobilization of the spine with a brace or collar may be necessary in the interim.

The lateral view should be inspected for alignment (Fig. 11–2A). Lines drawn along

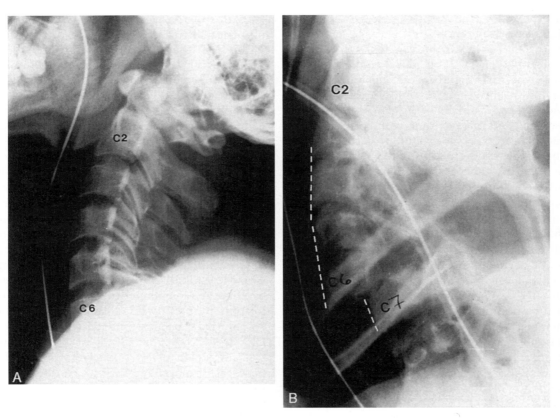

Figure 11–1. C6-C7 subluxation. *(A)* Initial crosstable lateral view of the cervical spine shows normal alignment to C6. *(B)* However, a swimmer's view obtained to visualize the lower cervical spine and cervicothoracic junction discloses a nearly complete anterior subluxation of the body of C6 on C7 in this paraplegic patient. (From Mettler FA: Essentials of Radiology. Philadelphia, WB Saunders, 1996, p 273.)

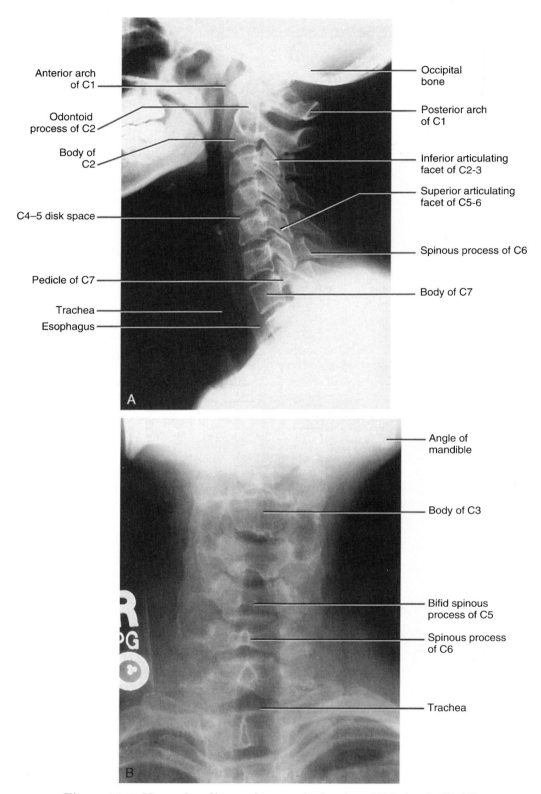

Figure 11–2. Normal radiographs, cervical spine. *(A)* Lateral, *(B)* AP.

Illustration continued on following page

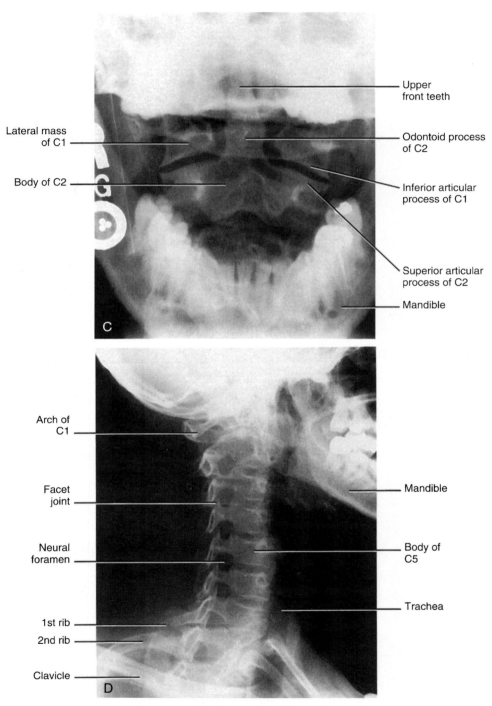

Figure 11–2 *Continued (C)* Odontoid, and *(D)* oblique views. (From Mettler FA: Essentials of Radiology. Philadelphia, WB Saunders, 1996, pp 259, 262, 265.)

the anterior cortex, posterior body cortex, and posterior lamina/anterior spinous process junction should be smooth (Fig. 11–3). The prevertebral soft tissue planes of the upper cervical spine are normally close to the spine, and a fat plane is often visible anterior to the vertebral bodies. Swelling of the prevertebral soft tissues or displacement of the fat plane may be indicative of trauma and possible fracture. The prevertebral tissues are normally not more than 4 mm thick at the C3 level under standard imaging conditions. Magnification that is associated with portable radiography can increase the apparent soft tissue thickness. Disc space widening and focal kyphotic angulation also indicate levels of injury. Disc space narrowing may occur with acute injury, but it is also a very common degenerative change. Fractures may be manifested as lucency, increased density if bones are crushed or overlap, or an abnormal contour.

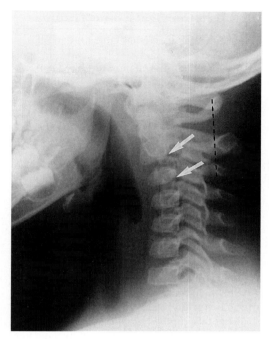

Figure 11–4. Cervical spine pseudosubluxation in a child. Lateral radiograph in an infant shows apparent subluxation of the C2 body anterior to the C3 vertebral body *(arrows)*. However, the spinolaminar line *(dashed black line)* is normal, and the appearance is normal for a child of this age.

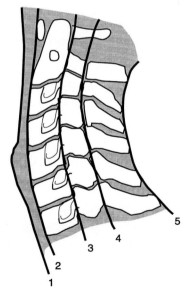

Figure 11–3. Normal lateral cervical spine. Diagram of lines to evaluate alignment of the lateral cervical spine. There should be a smooth curve as illustrated, without focal angulation (kyphosis) or stepoff. Indicated at (1) is the anterior margin of the prevertebral soft tissues; at (2) is the anterior spinal line (anterior margin of the vertebral bodies); at (3) is the posterior spinal line (posterior margin of the vertebral bodies); at (4) is the spinolaminar line, and at (5) is the spinous process line.

Children normally have greater ligamentous laxity than adults. Apparent anterior displacement of the body of C2 relative to C3 is a common finding in children and is usually normal. Even so, the anterior margin of the spinous processes from C1 through C3 (spinolaminar line) should fall along a straight line (Fig. 11–4).

The lateral margins of the cervical spine have a smooth, undulating course on a normal AP view (Fig. 11–2*B*). The spinous processes lie near the midline without abrupt change in position from one level to the next. On the normal odontoid view, the outer margins of the lateral masses of C1 align with the outer edge of the C2 body (Fig. 11–2*C*).

COMMON CERVICAL SPINE INJURIES

Typical abnormalities in some common fractures are presented here. A more complete

TABLE 11–1. **Cervical Spine Trauma**

Injuries of the cervicocranial junction and atlas (C1)
  Atlanto-occipital dissociation (usually fatal)
  Jefferson burst fracture of C1 (axial load injury)
  Avulsion fracture of the anterior arch of C1
  Posterior arch fracture of C1 (hyperextension injury)
  Transverse ligament rupture or avulsion
  Rotatory subluxation
Fractures of the axis (C2)
  Dens fracture (also termed type II odontoid fracture)
  Avulsion fracture of the tip of the dens (also termed type I odontoid fracture; rare and associated with other major injuries)
  C2 body fracture, type 1: coronally oriented through posterior body
  C2 body fracture, type 2: predominantly sagittally oriented, "burst" (axial load injury)
  C2 body fracture, type 3: horizontally oriented rostral (also termed type III odontoid fracture)
  Traumatic spondylolisthesis (hangman's fracture)
  Lamina fracture
  Extension teardrop fracture
C3 through C7 injuries
  Spinous process (clay-shoveler's) fracture
  Flexion sprain
  Compression fracture
  Bilateral facet dislocation
  Flexion teardrop fracture
  Unilateral facet dislocation or facet fracture
  Pillar fracture
  Lamina fracture
  Hyperextension-dislocation
  Hyperextension fracture-dislocation
  Burst fracture

listing of cervical spine injuries is given in Table 11–1. Many variations occur. The reader who deals regularly with spine trauma is encouraged to study texts dedicated to this subject.

Cervicocranial Disruption

Dislocation at the cervicocranial junction requires strong forces to tear the multiple ligaments that attach the spine to the skull. Such injuries are usually fatal. Infrequently, however, patients survive. Dislocation can take place in either anterior or posterior directions, and distraction may also occur. Normally, a line drawn along the

posterior margin of the clivus should point to the tip or posterior portion of the top of the dens. Alteration of this relationship is an important clue to occipitoatlantal dissociation. A variety of measurements have been proposed to show relationships between the foramen magnum, C1, and C2. Such measurements may be useful but are limited because of the different directions in which dislocation may occur.

Fractures of C1

The atlas (the C1 vertebra) has a unique ring-like shape without a centrum (body). Axial loading injuries, such as diving accidents, can cause a Jefferson (C1 burst) fracture, in which the ring is fractured in several locations, both anteriorly and posteriorly (Fig. 11–5). Common radiographic abnormalities include lateral displacement of the lateral masses of C1 on the odontoid view and prevertebral soft tissue swelling. CT shows the fractures well. The transverse atlantal ligament is occasionally ruptured or avulsed, representing an additional threat to stability. Transverse ligament rupture can also accompany other fractures or can occur as an isolated but serious injury. Lateral displacement of the lateral masses of C1 relative to C2 of more than 7 mm as

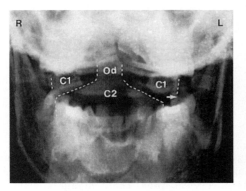

Figure 11–5. Jefferson (C1) burst fracture. On the openmouth AP view, the left lateral mass of C1 extends laterally beyond the margin of C2 *(arrow)*. The space between the medial margin of the C1 left lateral mass and the odontoid process is widened. (From Mettler FA: Essentials of Radiology. Philadelphia, WB Saunders, 1996, p 266.)

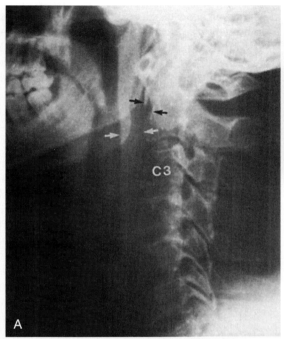

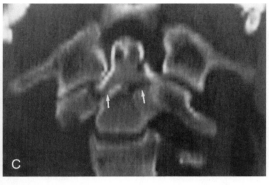

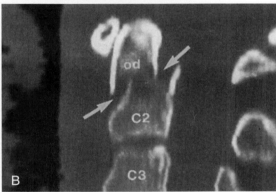

Figure 11–6. Fracture through the base of the odontoid process. *(A)* Cross-table lateral radiograph of the cervical spine shows anterior displacement of the dens relative to the body of C2, with a fragment visible anteriorly *(black arrows)*. There is prevertebral soft tissue swelling *(white arrows)*. (From Mettler FA: Essentials of Radiology. Philadelphia, WB Saunders, 1996, p 266.) *(B* and *C)* Reformatted sagittal *(B)* and coronal *(C)* images from axial CT scan demonstrate that the fracture plane *(arrows)* is primarily at the base of the odontoid process, through the body of C2.

seen on an AP view (sum of both sides) is likely to be associated with transverse ligament instability, although MRI evidence of ligament disruption is more reliable as a clinical predictor. Fractures of only the posterior arch of C1 are caused by hyperextension and, without other injuries, pose little threat to stability.

Fractures of C2

Multiple types of fractures can occur at C2 (the axis). Fractures can occur through the odontoid process. Nondisplaced or minimally displaced odontoid fractures can be quite difficult to detect. Fractures below the base of the odontoid process are also common. These are actually horizontal fractures through the body of C2 and have a better overall healing rate than dens fractures (Fig. 11–6). Another abnormality that involves the dens is the os odontoideum, in which the dens constitutes a separate bone that is not attached to the body of C2. It can radiographically resemble a dens fracture. Although there is disagreement regarding the etiology of the os odontoideum, it represents a threat to spinal stability.

Axial loading forces can cause fractures that are roughly sagittally oriented through the body of C2 if the ring of C1 remains intact. The fracture begins adjacent to the

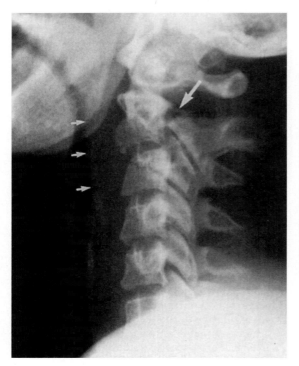

Figure 11–7. Hangman's fracture (traumatic spondylolisthesis). Lateral cervical spine radiograph shows lucency posterior to the C2 vertebral body (through the pars interarticularis *(large arrow)* and prevertebral soft tissue swelling *(small arrows)*. A tiny fracture fragment is also present at the anterior inferior corner of the C2 body. (From Mettler FA: Essentials of Radiology. Philadelphia, WB Saunders, 1996, p 268.)

base of the dens and is obliquely sagittal in orientation. Displacement and neurologic injury are common.

Several different mechanisms can lead to a third type of C2 body fracture, in which there is a coronally-oriented fracture through the posterior aspect of the C2 body.

Avulsion at the attachment of the anterior longitudinal ligament is responsible for extension teardrop fractures, which appear as a triangular fragment at the anterior inferior aspect of the C2 vertebral body.

Traumatic spondylolisthesis of C2 is often referred to as the *hangman's fracture,* although the mechanism is hyperextension. Fractures occur through the pars interarticularis of C2 bilaterally (Fig. 11–7). Displacement ranges from minimal to severe, with

the likelihood of complications greater with increased fracture displacement. Because the spinal canal is usually not significantly narrowed, the patient is often spared neurologic injury. Hyperextension can also cause laminar fractures.

Fractures of the Lower Cervical Spine: Burst Fractures

The C3 through C7 vertebral bodies are morphologically similar, and they differ from the unique shapes of C1 and C2. If axial loading forces extend into this region, burst fractures may occur. Forces transmitted through the intervertebral disc, downward into the centrum, lead to disruption of the vertebral body (Fig. 11–8). The degree of comminution and fragment displacement is variable, and disruption and narrowing of the spinal canal often lead to spinal cord damage. When this fracture occurs, overall

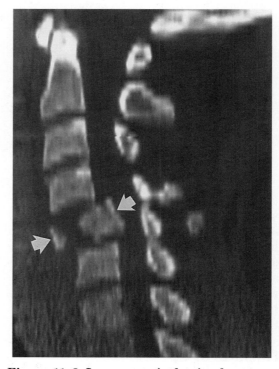

Figure 11–8. Lower cervical spine burst fracture. Sagittal reformation view from a CT scan of a patient who suffered a burst fracture of C5 after an axial-loading mechanism injury. There is major displacement of the fragments of the vertebral body *(arrows).*

alignment of the cervical spine on the lateral view is generally straight, and a prominent sagittal component of the fracture is often visible on AP views or CT. CT is advantageous for evaluation of bone fragments in the spinal canal. Posterior element fractures often accompany burst fractures.

Fractures of the Lower Cervical Spine: Flexion Injuries

Flexion injuries often leave the spine in a flexed position on the lateral view. Focal kyphosis and widening of the facet joints and laminae on the lateral radiograph are often signs of flexion sprain. This injury, which is caused by damage to the posterior ligaments, can lead to delayed instability (Fig. 11–9*A*).

Greater applied force, with the neck flexed, can lead to several types of fractures that are usually accompanied by ligamentous injury. Compression fractures are recognized by greater loss of height of the vertebral body anteriorly than posteriorly and by buckling of the cortex of the anterior vertebral body and superior endplate (Fig. 11–9*B,C*).

Disruption of the facet joints in flexion can cause bilateral facet dislocation, which is an unstable injury (Fig. 11–10). The facet component of the superior vertebra normally lies posterior to the facet component from the inferior vertebra at the facet joint, which is a relationship referred to as *shingling* (Fig. 11–2*D*). The joint is widened in bilateral facet dislocation, and the upper facets lie above (or anterior to) the lower facets. The upper vertebral body at the level of injury is displaced anteriorly, usually a distance of half or more of the vertebral body width. There is a significant risk of spinal cord compression.

The patient with a flexion teardrop fracture is usually neurologically devastated, typically exhibiting a complete myelopathy and an anterior spinal cord syndrome. The anterior spinal cord syndrome is associated with a complete loss of motor function below the level of injury and an accompanying partial sensory loss (with some sparing of posterior column function). A characteristic appearance is observed on the lateral radiograph, with a large, anterior, inferior vertebral body fracture fragment and kyphotic angulation of the spine.

Sudden flexion against strained muscles can lead to avulsion of one or more spinous processes (clay-shoveler's fracture) (Fig. 11–11). This fracture alone is of relatively minor significance but can accompany other spine injuries.

Fractures of the Lower Cervical Spine: Rotational Injuries

A combination of flexion and rotation force vectors can lead to unilateral facet dislocation, sometimes referred to as a *locked* or *perched* facet. On the lateral view, the upper vertebral body at the level of injury is displaced anteriorly less than half the distance of a vertebral body, and an abrupt change in the appearance of the posterior elements occurs at the level of dislocation (Fig. 11–12). Because of rotation, on the lateral projection the upper spine presents the appearance commonly observed on an oblique view, and the lower cervical spine appears as it is usually observed on a lateral view. The facets at the level of the dislocation have a bowtie configuration on the lateral view. Rotation is indicated on the AP view by an abrupt change in position of the spinous processes (Fig. 11–12*C*). Associated fractures of the articular processes are also common with these injuries, and are often best detected with CT.

Rotation and hyperextension can cause pillar fractures. These fractures of the articular mass on one side can be difficult to identify by plain films. The pillar view shows the articular mass well, but this projection is seldom part of the routine cervical spine film series. CT is more helpful. Fractures that either isolate or extend into the articular mass, along with associated ligamentous injury, can cause delayed instability and rotational injury.

Fractures of the Lower Cervical Spine: Extension Injuries

Hyperextension can lead to laminar fractures, the hangman's fracture of C2 described earlier, and extension teardrop fractures. Hyperextension-dislocation is a

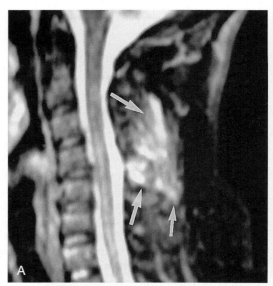

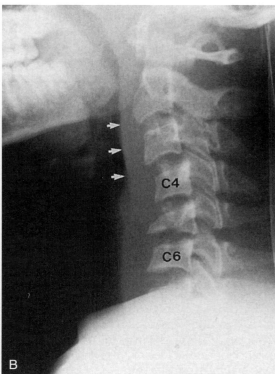

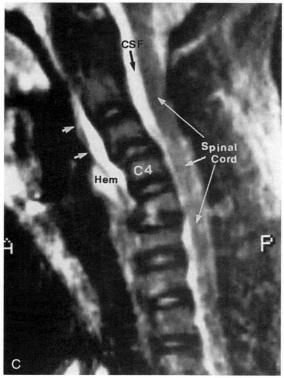

Figure 11–9. Lower cervical spine flexion injuries. Flexion sprain may occur without fractures. *(A)* Sagittal T2-weighted MRI of a woman who was in a motor vehicle accident shows high signal intensity of edema and/or hemorrhage in the posterior soft tissues *(arrows),* with the deepest extent in the C4-5 interspinous ligament region. There is mild kyphosis. Although there were no fractures, later flexion radiograph confirmed instability at C4-5. With greater force, often both fractures and ligamentous injury occur. *(B)* Lateral radiograph of another trauma patient shows anterior wedging of the C5 vertebral body. There is widening of the posterior elements between C5 and C6. Prevertebral soft tissue swelling is present *(arrows).* *(C)* Sagittal T2WI from MRI shows the fractured vertebral body, and high signal intensity in the prevertebral *(arrows,* hemorrhage) and posterior soft tissues. *(B* and *C* from Mettler FA: Essentials of Radiology. Philadelphia, WB Saunders, 1996, p 269.)

serious injury caused by disruption of the anterior longitudinal ligament and an intervertebral disc. The plain film appearance can be subtle. Radiographic signs include diffuse prevertebral soft tissue swelling with loss of cervical lordosis, widening of the disc space, and occasionally a thin anterior avulsion of an inferior endplate. The most common clinical condition caused by hyperextension-dislocation is the central spinal cord syndrome, in which motor loss is greater in the upper extremities than in lower extremities. The central spinal cord syndrome can also follow another type of hyperextension injury when degenerative changes are present. In this circumstance, the spinal cord may be transiently pinched between osteophytes and ligamentum flavum during hyperextension.

Hyperextension fracture-dislocation is a very serious and unstable injury. The cervical spine assumes a seemingly paradoxical

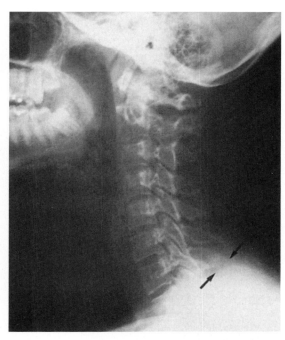

Figure 11–11. Clay-shoveler's fracture. An avulsion fracture of the spinous process of C7 is visible on this lateral radiograph of the cervical spine *(arrows)*. (From Mettler FA: Essentials of Radiology. Philadelphia, WB Saunders, 1996, p 272.)

flexed position on the lateral view in this type of fracture.

Cautions Regarding Cervical Spine Injuries

Many combinations and variations of these general fractures may occur. *More than one fracture is common in an injured cervical spine, and identification of one fracture should prompt a search for others.* Fractures can occur at different levels of the spine, occasionally at some distance, with intervening normal vertebra.

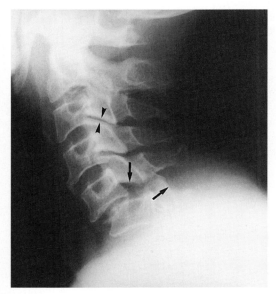

Figure 11–10. Bilateral facet dislocation. Lateral cervical spine radiograph of a man who fell off a bridge shows bilateral facet dislocation at C5-6. There is greater than 50 percent anterior displacement of C5 on C6. Space between the posterior elements is widened at that level. The normal shingle-like relationship of the facets (e.g., *arrowheads* at C3-4) is disrupted at C5-6 (*arrows* point to facets that should articulate).

THORACIC AND LUMBAR FRACTURES

Lateral and AP projections are routinely obtained in radiographic evaluation of the thoracic and lumbar segments of the spine. The

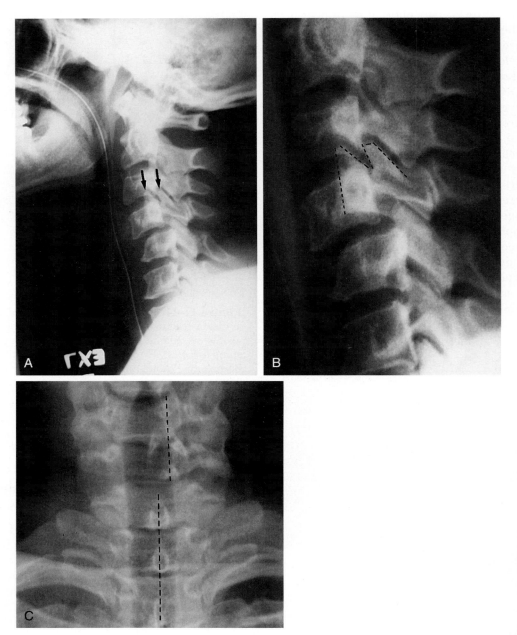

Figure 11–12. Unilateral facet dislocation. *(A)* Lateral view of the cervical spine. The C4 vertebral body is displaced anteriorly less than one-half of its width relative to C5. The upper cervical spine has a rotated or oblique orientation, and the lower cervical spine has a straight lateral orientation. At C4, both facets are visible *(arrows)*. The more anterior facet is dislocated on C5. *(B)* The "bowtie" appearance at the level of dislocation is visible on a magnified view *(dotted lines)*. *(C)* AP view of another patient with unilateral facet dislocation shows rotation above C6-C7, which is manifested by an abrupt change in the alignment of the spinous processes *(dashed lines)*.

alignment of the margins of the vertebral bodies should be smooth in both views. Acute thoracic fractures are often accompanied by a paraspinous hematoma, which can be visualized on an AP view. Transverse process fractures of the lumbar spine can be detected by AP views. Although of little mechanical significance, they serve as evidence of trauma and should alert one to the possibility of other fractures and of soft tissue injuries.

Compression fractures are fairly common in the thoracic and lumbar portions of the spine (Fig. 11–13). The thoracolumbar junction is especially prone to such injury. As with cervical compression fractures, loss of anterior vertebral body height (greater than posterior) is present on the lateral radiograph.

Burst fractures can also occur in the thoracic or lumbar spine. The risk of neurologic damage is related to the degree of bone displacement. Even if the spinal cord is intact, stabilization may be necessary.

Flexion-distraction injuries can lead to a Chance fracture (Fig. 11–14). This horizontal fracture through the vertebral body extends posteriorly into the neural arch. The fracture typically occurs in the upper lumbar vertebra. It is especially common in motor vehicle accidents when the patient's body is flexed over a lap-type seatbelt without a shoulder harness. Plain films demonstrate a fracture line involving the pedicles in addition to a vertebral body fracture.

Fracture-dislocations of the thoracic and lumbar spine result from severe forces and frequently lead to spinal cord compression or transection, and paraplegia. Plain films show the disruption, and CT can be helpful for operative planning.

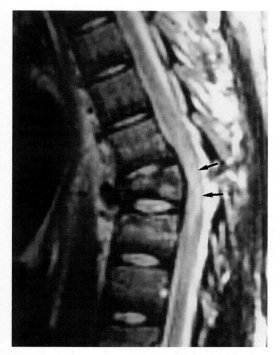

Figure 11–13. Compression fracture and spinal cord edema. MRI of an 18-year-old who was in a motor vehicle accident. Sagittal T2WI shows compression fracture of a midthoracic vertebral body, narrowing of the spinal canal, and high signal intensity within the spinal cord *(arrows)*. The patient was paraplegic.

MRI IN SPINE TRAUMA

MRI is gaining an increasingly important role in the evaluation of spine trauma. Some specific diagnostic areas in which MRI can be of benefit are listed below. The list is not inclusive, and additional research on the effective integration of MRI into trauma imaging can be expected.

1. *Evaluation of the spinal cord.* Spinal cord compression and displacement are well demonstrated on sagittal images (see Figs. 11–9, 11–13). Evidence of spinal cord damage has been shown to have prognostic value. Small areas of edema, extensive edema, and intramedullary hemorrhage have increasingly worse prognoses.

2. *Evaluation of intervertebral discs.* Traumatic disc disruption or herniation of the nucleus pulposus (HNP) is not observed with plain films and is shown much better with MRI than with CT. It is a possible cause of neurologic worsening after reduction of a fracture or dislocation. Recognition of a traumatic HNP therefore may alter surgical planning. Because disc degeneration is common, incidental HNP may be observed, and clinical correlation with MRI findings is mandatory.

3. *Detection of ligamentous injury.* MRI is

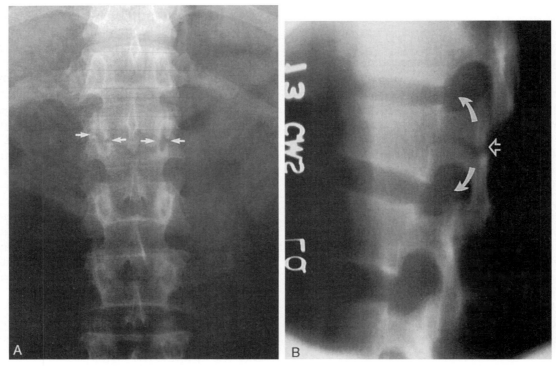

Figure 11–14. Chance fracture. *(A)* AP radiograph of a patient who was wearing a lap-type seat belt (and no shoulder harness) during an accident shows lucencies through the pedicles of L2 *(arrows).* *(B)* Lateral tomogram confirms posterior element fractures *(open arrow).* There is also anterior vertebral body compression. *Curved arrows* depict distraction forces. (From Mettler FA: Essentials of Radiology. Philadelphia, WB Saunders, 1996, p 284.)

sensitive to soft tissue injury in the acute care setting and can be beneficial in identifying patients whose injuries constitute an increased risk of instability. Major soft tissue injury with no fracture or with minimally displaced fractures can still be significant.

4. *Vascular injury.* Vertebral artery damage and occlusion may occur with cervical spine fractures, especially when fractures involve the foramen transversarium. MRI is a noninvasive method of imaging blood flow (or lack of flow).

5. *The problem patient.* MRI may be very helpful in some challenging diagnostic settings. For example, clinical evaluation is often quite limited in patients with head injury or in those who are otherwise unable to communicate. The patient with significant neck pain and normal x-ray study results may have significant nonosseous injuries. When confounding factors such as

severe degenerative change or arthritis make it difficult to determine whether an acute major injury has occurred, MRI can provide useful additional information.

6. *Complications of spinal trauma.* Chronic sequelae of spinal cord damage (for example, myelomalacia, cysts, and syrinx formation) are best visualized with MRI (Fig. 11–15). If surgery is performed, MRI can be used to follow the outcome of such treatment.

CONCLUSIONS

Imaging of spinal trauma should always take place in the context of the clinical findings. The various imaging modalities available for acute spinal trauma have inherently different characteristics. Under-

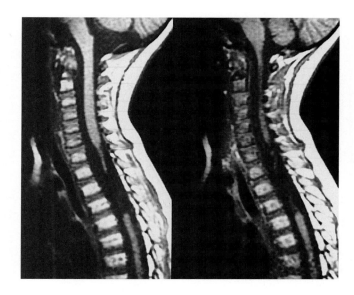

Figure 11–15. Spinal cord atrophy after trauma. MRI (cervical T1WI, two adjacent slices) of a 1-year-old infant who had been in an automobile accident 2 months previously and was now paraplegic. Radiographs of the cervical spine were normal. There is severe atrophy of the lower cervical and upper thoracic spinal cord. Flexion, distraction, and ischemia have all been hypothesized as possible causes of spinal cord injury without radiographic abnormality.

standing the most common imaging appearance and the complementary nature of imaging studies can help guide the appropriate use of imaging following acute trauma. The purposes of imaging tests during evaluation of spine trauma are to detect occult but dangerous injuries, to aid in preventing the worsening of injuries, and to assist in monitoring treatment and recovery.

12

Nontraumatic Acquired
Disorders of the Spine

Acquired disorders of the spine other than trauma (which is addressed in the previous chapter) are discussed in this chapter. Degenerative diseases of the spine, especially those resulting in low back and neck pain, are very common clinical problems. Other acquired conditions are less common but also carry significant morbidity. Infectious and other inflammatory conditions, neoplasms of the spine, vascular disorders, and demyelinating diseases are examples. Various conditions may result in a central fluid-filled cavity, or syrinx, of the spinal cord, and the differential diagnosis of this entity is also presented.

DEGENERATIVE DISEASES OF THE SPINE

Low back pain is extremely common and is a major cause of disability and lost work time. Imaging of the lumbosacral spine is thus part of an important and complex medical decision-making process. Neck pain and other sequelae of degenerative diseases of the spine and the intervertebral discs are also common and, therefore, important. Because various techniques are available for imaging the spine, it is very useful to understand the strengths and limitations of these

techniques to incorporate them appropriately into diagnostic algorithms.

Clinical Features

Back or neck pain may occur with or without radiation into the extremities. The hallmark of radiculopathy (irritation of a nerve root) is pain referred into the arm and hand from a cervical source or into the leg and foot from a lumbar source. Radicular pain may be accompanied by signs of sensory loss, weakness, atrophy, or loss of reflexes. Compression of the spinal cord and myelopathy may result in weakness of the legs and sometimes arms, hyperreflexia, sensory loss (particularly to pain and temperature on the trunk or loss of position and vibration sense in the extremities), or bladder and sphincter abnormalities. Focal neck or back pain can be caused by various disease processes including ligamentous or soft tissue strain, infection, malignancy, or trauma. Characterization of the pain as local or radicular helps in formulating a differential diagnosis and choosing the best imaging procedure. Guidelines exist to help determine when to order an imaging study of the cervical, thoracic, or lumbosacral spine.

Radiographic Techniques

X-ray-based techniques (plain films and CT) are superior to MRI for visualizing bones and other calcified structures. Plain films are thus helpful for the evaluation of alignment abnormalities (including *spondylolisthesis*, or displacement of one vertebral body relative to an adjacent vertebral body), *spondylolysis* (a bony defect through the pars interarticularis), and degenerative changes (sometimes referred as to as *spondylosis*) (Fig. 12–1). Oblique views of the lumbar spine add considerable radiation exposure and often add little diagnostic information, especially for the routine evaluation of back pain. Oblique views of the cervical spine add useful information about neural foraminal narrowing. CT provides information regarding the size of the spinal canal and the extent of degenerative facet changes. The intervertebral discs are visible on CT, although not as clearly as on MRI. Although CT may be used as an initial screening test for significant disc hernia-

tion, MRI is generally considered to be superior.

MRI and Degenerative Spine Disease

MRI has distinct advantages over CT for evaluation of degenerative spine disease, especially if surgery is being considered. Many consider MRI the imaging study of choice for the evaluation of significant and persistent low back pain, especially that with radiculopathy. MRI is more sensitive than CT for evaluation of soft tissues. This includes not only the spinal cord and discs, but the marrow spaces as well. On the other hand, cortical bone, which has little MR-visible signal, is poorly visualized. The normal intervertebral disc has high signal intensity centrally on conventional spin-echo T2-weighted images. With aging, however, changes in proteoglycan content lead to loss of signal intensity. Such signal loss alone is expected with aging and commonly occurs at one or two intervertebral disc levels as early as young adulthood. This is of doubtful clinical significance as an isolated finding.

Disc Protrusion and Herniation

Herniation of the nucleus pulposus (HNP) is a treatable cause of back pain and neurologic symptoms (Figs. 12–2 through 12–5). Disc impingement on a nerve may lead to radiculopathy. In the lumbar spine, this most commonly affects the nerve that is to exit via the next most caudal intervertebral foramen (see Figs. 12–2, 12–4). For example, a left paracentral HNP at L4-L5, if symptomatic, most commonly causes a left L5 radiculopathy. However, a far lateral HNP that causes narrowing of the neural foramen can affect the next higher nerve root (in the earlier example, the L4 nerve root) (see Figs. 12–2, 12–5). A severe herniation with a significant narrowing of the spinal canal can affect multiple nerves.

Although myelography with CT has been the gold standard in the past for diagnosis of HNP, its role is now significantly limited. CT and MRI can both demonstrate HNP, but MRI can provide images directly in multiple planes. Furthermore, it can demonstrate intervertebral disc pathology (see

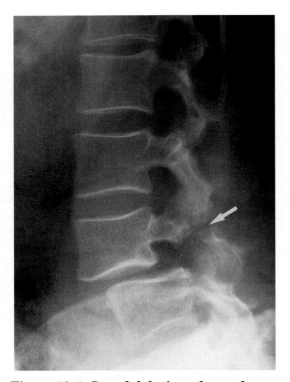

Figure 12–1. Spondylolysis and spondylolisthesis. Lateral radiograph of the lumbar spine shows grade 2 spondylolisthesis (anterior displacement) of the L4 vertebral body on L5. The cause is spondylolysis (defects through the pars interarticularis) of L4 *(arrow).*

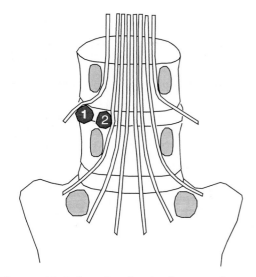

Figure 12–2. Levels of spinal nerve damage from disc protrusions. Diagram of a posterior view of nerve roots of the lower lumbar spine and sacrum. A far *lateral* disc herniation (1) affects the exiting nerve *at* that level. A *paracentral* HNP (2), which is more common, usually affects the nerve roots *below* that level.

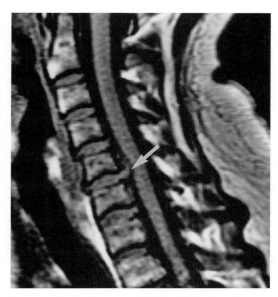

Figure 12–3. Cervical HNP. MRI of a 35-year-old woman with neck and right arm pain. Sagittal T1WI shows posterior disc protrusion *(arrow)* with slight superior extension at the C5-6 level.

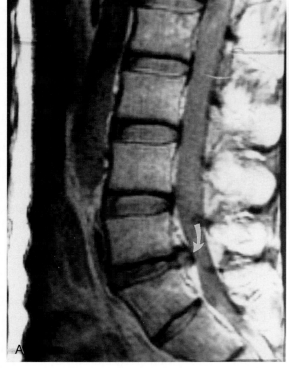

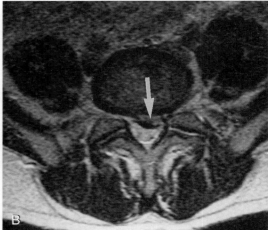

Figure 12–4. Lumbar HNP. MRI of a 33-year-old man with back pain. *(A)* Sagittal T2WI shows narrowing of the L4-L5 intervertebral disc height, decreased signal intensity relative to the other disks, and posterior protrusion of disc material *(arrow)*. *(B)* On axial T2WI, the HNP *(arrow)* is in part bright and narrows the left side of the spinal canal.

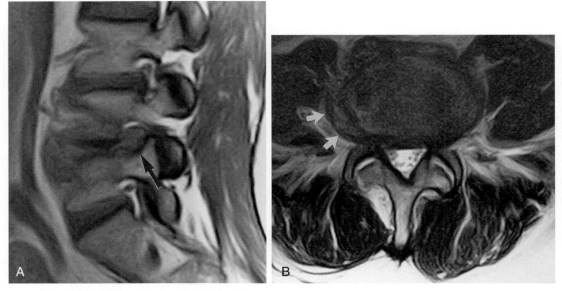

Figure 12–5. Lateral disc protrusion. *(A)* On a right parasagittal T1WI, abnormal soft tissue is present within the L4-L5 neural foramen *(arrow),* replacing most of the fat that is normally present. At levels above and below, there is a normal appearance of the spinal nerve exiting the foramen just inferior to the pedicle, with fat filling the remainder of the foramen. *(B)* The far lateral disc protrusion or herniation *(arrows)* is visible on an axial T2WI.

Figs. 12–3, 12–4, 12–5). An HNP is an extension of the disc that has "herniated" into the spinal canal. However, the clear identification of the herniation of the nucleus pulposus and the status of the posterior longitudinal ligament are pathologic diagnoses that cannot be determined with certainty by imaging. Therefore, it is important that there is clear communication between the radiologist and the referring clinician regarding the imaging results. For example, a broad-based disc protrusion is important to differentiate from an extruded fragment with a narrow base of attachment to the disc. The latter is very likely to represent an HNP, whereas the significance of the former is less certain. A potential pitfall is the sequestered fragment. Such a fragment can migrate either rostrally or caudally (with respect to the parent disc level). Migration is extremely important to recognize because it can alter the surgical approach.

The presence of conjoined nerve roots, a congenital variant, may simulate pathology such as HNP. It is fairly common, especially at S1-S2 and L5-S1, for two nerve roots to share a common proximal sheath before separating to exit through their respective neural foramina. This results in asymmetry in the appearance of the thecal sac on axial imaging (Fig. 12–6). It is important to recognize the benign nature of this asymmetry and not confuse it with disc protrusion. The presence of conjoined nerve roots can also have clinical significance, because the more rostral of the two conjoined nerve roots takes a more caudal, and more acute, course than usual within the neural foramen. Pathology of the foramen, such as osteophytes or a far lateral disc protrusion, may thus impinge on a conjoined nerve root that might otherwise be unaffected. Moreover, if surgery is considered, the surgeon should be made aware of the anomalous course of a nerve root that may lie within the surgical field.

Spinal Stenosis

Spinal stenosis is often multifactorial in origin. Etiologies include acquired degenerative changes such as osteophyte formation, disc disease, facet arthropathy, and accompanying prominence (hypertrophy) of the

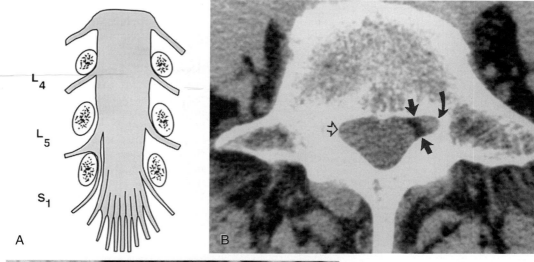

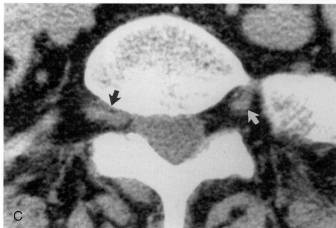

Figure 12–6. Conjoined nerve roots. *(A)* The normal pattern of nerve roots exiting inferior to the pedicles is depicted on the *right* side of the diagram. Conjoined nerve roots are depicted on the *left* side of diagram (L5 and S1). *(B)* Axial nonenhanced CT at the level of L5 shows asymmetry in the lateral recesses. Normal fat *(solid straight arrows)* is present around the *left* L5 nerve *(curved arrow).* Uniform soft tissue density extends from the thecal sac to the right lateral recess, where the *right* L5 nerve lies *(open arrow).* Proximal nerve sheaths of the *right* L5 and S1 nerves are conjoined. *(C)* At a lower level, just below the pedicles, the *left* L5 nerve has already exited the foramen *(white arrow).* The *right* L5 nerve *(black arrow)* lies more caudally within the foramen, and is therefore more medial at this level.

ligamentum flavum. Occasionally, a congenitally narrow spinal canal (short pedicles) contributes to spinal stenosis. Clinical findings in spinal stenosis typically include back pain and neurogenic claudication. The latter must be distinguished from claudication of vascular origin. CT and MRI are both capable of demonstrating the pathologic structural findings (Fig. 12–7). More than one spinal level is usually involved. Stenosis may occur centrally or in the lateral recess of the spinal canal. Measurements of the spinal canal may be helpful. For example, less than 12 mm anteroposterior (AP) diameter in the lumbar spine is abnormal. However, assessment must include a description of multiple factors, including the size of the central canal, lateral recesses, and neural foramina; presence of distortion of the thecal sac; and reasons for the stenosis.

Calcification or ossification of the posterior longitudinal ligament (OPLL) is an uncommon condition that can cause cervical spinal stenosis and myelopathy. It was originally described in Japan, with about 2 percent prevalence in that country, but it is not limited to the Far East. The calcification may be diffuse (continuous) or segmental

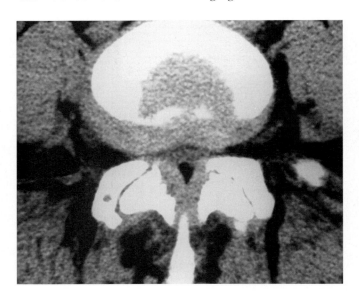

Figure 12–7. Lumbar spinal stenosis. The spinal canal is significantly narrowed at the L4-L5 level, as seen on a noncontrasted lumbar spine CT scan. The pedicles cause this canal to be congenitally somewhat narrow, and there is further spinal canal encroachment from facet hypertrophy, prominent ligamentum flavum, and a diffusely bulging disc.

(discontinuous) and can be identified on plain film or CT (Fig. 12–8). MRI is less reliable for demonstration of OPLL.

Imaging of the Postoperative Spine

Postoperatively, imaging of the spine poses special problems, especially in the lumbar spine. In addition to the expected bony changes, often there is extensive soft tissue change related to surgery (for example, discectomy) and granulation tissue or scar. In the first few weeks following surgery, the appearance of soft tissue changes may be impossible to separate from disc herniation. The presence of metal creates artifacts on both CT and MRI. Not only do metallic implants cause such artifacts, but it is common for tiny pieces of metal (resulting from drilling with high speed burrs that contact other metal objects) to cause artifacts on MRI, even if the metal is not visible by x-ray examination. The increasing use of titanium spine hardware facilitates the acquisition of MRI without major artifact.

Intravenous contrast material is often very helpful in separating scar from residual or recurrent disc herniation. Scar or granulation tissue, which may be observed for years following surgery, typically enhances promptly (within 5 minutes) following intravenous (IV) contrast material administration. Although disc material can

enhance on MRI because of vascularization or diffusion, this phenomenon occurs more slowly and is generally observed only with delayed imaging (20 minutes or more after contrast material administration). MRI or CT of the postoperative lumbar spine is therefore performed immediately following IV contrast material administration (Figs. 12–9, 12–10).

Integrating Imaging Studies into Clinical Management

The imaging of degenerative spine disease should be planned with treatment implications and expected clinical outcomes in mind. Because degenerative changes of the spine are extremely common, asymptomatic or only minimally symptomatic changes are found frequently in the adult population. Therefore, careful correlation with clinical findings is mandatory before attaching significance to imaging findings of spine disease. Moreover, many patients with back or neck pain improve with nonoperative, conservative medical rehabilitation therapy. Imaging should be performed only after an appropriate interval (generally, after at least 6 weeks of conservative therapy) and when treatment may be altered by the imaging results. The presence of neurologic deficits may warrant a more expeditious use of imaging studies. There is currently a

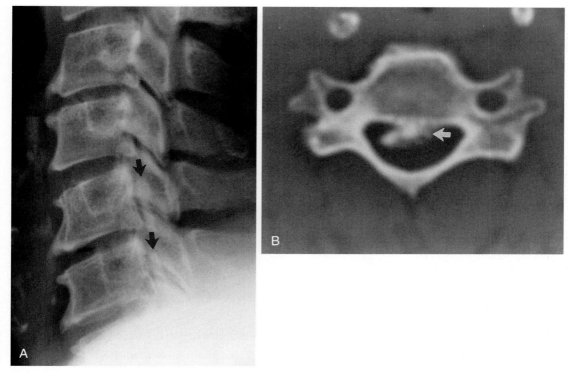

Figure 12–8. Ossification of the posterior longitudinal ligament. *(A)* Abnormal calcification *(arrows)* is present dorsal to the lower cervical vertebral bodies on a lateral cervical radiograph of a man with symptoms of cervical spinal stenosis. *(B)* Axial CT scan also demonstrates the calcification in the region of the posterior longitudinal ligament *(arrow)*. (From Jahnke RW, Hart BL. Cervical stenosis, spondylosis, and herniated disc disease. Radiol Clin North Am 29(4):779, 1991.)

great deal of interest and investigation into the timing of and use of the most appropriate imaging studies for these very common conditions.

INFECTIOUS AND INFLAMMATORY CONDITIONS

Infection in and around the spine can spread to involve adjacent structures, including bone, disc, muscles and other soft tissues, the epidural space, thecal sac, and spinal cord. Imaging is used to identify the extent of infection, as well as to provide information regarding related complications, such as abscess formation.

Vertebral and Intervertebral Disc Infection

Discitis (infection of the disc space) or spondylitis (infection or inflammation of the ver-

tebra) may arise from a variety of infectious origins. *Staphylococcus aureus* is the most common causative organism, but a variety of others cause infection, including *Salmonella, Escherichia coli,* and other gram-negative organisms; tuberculosis and brucellosis also occur. Risk factors include IV drug abuse, diabetes, and genitourinary infections. Hematogenous spread is thought to be the usual mechanism that starts infection in the spine. Infection generally begins in a subchondral location and then spreads to the disc space. Contiguous extension of infection to the marrow space and to the surrounding muscles and other paraspinous soft tissues, as well as to the epidural space, is possible. Subligamentous spread to adjacent vertebral levels is also common. Destruction of bone and disc lead to pain, spinal instability, kyphosis, and loss of height of the spine. Paraspinous abscess can result. Epidural abscess can lead to spinal cord

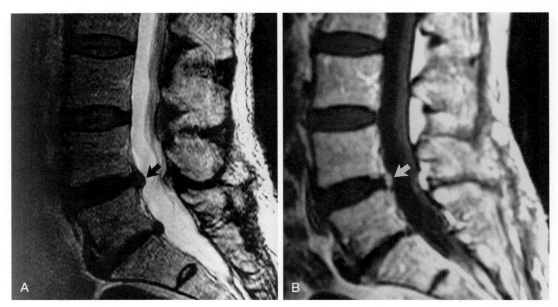

Figure 12–9. Postoperative spine MRI: scarring. Sagittal MRI of a woman with back pain and history of previous surgery at L4-L5. *(A)* A T2WI is strongly suggestive of recurrent or residual HNP at L4-L5 *(arrow)*. *(B)* However, after gadolinium administration (T1WI), the material at the posterior margin of the L4-L5 disc demonstrates intense and prompt enhancement *(arrow),* which is most consistent with scar or granulation tissue.

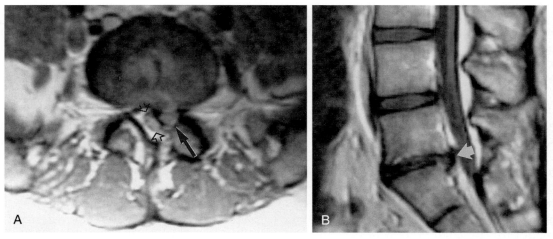

Figure 12–10. Postoperative spine MRI: recurrent disc herniation. *(A)* MRI (axial T2WI) of a young man with a history of previous disc surgery demonstrates deviation of the thecal sac *(open arrows)* to the right, and abnormal material in the left side of the spinal canal at the L5-S1 level *(solid arrow).* This could represent either recurrent herniation of disc material or scarring or granulation tissue. *(B)* However, unlike the case illustrated in Figure 12–9, there is no significant enhancement on post-gadolinium images *(arrow).*

compression and rapid neurologic impairment. Rupture into the thecal sac is a rare but potentially fatal complication, and thus epidural abscess represents a surgical emergency in most cases.

Early radiographic evidence of discitis includes endplate destruction and loss of disc height. With time, there is further bone destruction involving the vertebral bodies. Sclerosis occurs later, during the process of healing (Fig. 12–11). Radionuclide bone scans are more sensitive than plain radiographs, and they show abnormalities earlier than radiographs. CT can clearly display details of bone change and can also demonstrate paraspinous abscess (Fig. 12–11*B*).

MRI is very helpful for the evaluation of discitis and osteomyelitis, which are often associated. Osteomyelitis causes a pattern of decreased signal intensity on T1-weighted images and increased signal on T2-weighted images (Figs. 12–12, 12–13) in place of the normal marrow pattern that is largely dominated by fat signal intensity (see Fig. 10–1*A*). This MRI pattern of marrow replacement is nonspecific. Neoplasm or myeloproliferative disorders, for example, can cause a similar appearance (Fig. 12–14). However, neoplasm seldom crosses the disc space, whereas infection often does so.

Infected intervertebral discs also have al-tered signal. This can vary but is often heterogeneous (see Figs. 12–12, 12–13). The marrow space and the disc itself can show some enhancement with IV contrast material administration (see Fig. 12–12). The use of postcontrast T1-weighted magnetic resonance images alone may be deceptive and should be avoided, because enhancement can simulate the normal appearance of fat in the marrow. Fat suppression post-gadolinium and inversion recovery techniques can also be employed for the evaluation of bone marrow processes. Gadolinium administration is of greater benefit for demonstrating the presence and extent of epidural disease. Paraspinous inflammation can also be readily recognized on MRI (see Fig. 12–12).

There is considerable overlap in the imaging appearance from spinal infections caused by different organisms. Definitive diagnosis must rest on culture or biopsy. Nevertheless, spinal tuberculosis often causes extensive bone destruction and is associated with a prominent paraspinous soft tissue mass, whereas brucellosis is less often accompanied by paraspinous abscess.

Epidural Abscess

Epidural abscess may arise from either a hematogenous source or via direct inocula-

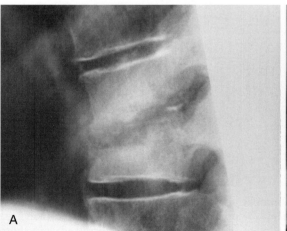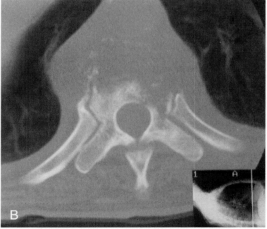

Figure 12–11. *Staphylococcus aureus* **spondylitis.** *(A)* Lateral thoracic spine radiograph shows disc space narrowing, end-plate destruction, and lytic process extending into the vertebral body. *(B)* Extensive bone destruction is also visible on CT.

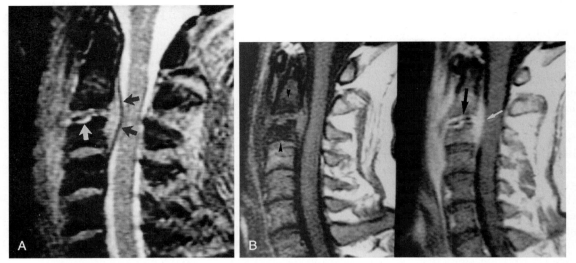

Figure 12–12. Cervical spondylitis, osteomyelitis, and epidural abscess in a drug abuser.
MRI of a man with neck pain and history of intravenous drug abuse. *(A)* Sagittal T2WI shows abnormal disc signal at C2-C3 *(white arrow),* disc space narrowing, increased signal intensity in the adjacent marrow, and an epidural mass dorsal to the vertebral bodies *(black arrows). (B)* T1WI before *(left)* and after *(right)* gadolinium contrast administration show marrow edema (low signal before contrast administration, *arrowheads)* and extensive enhancement of the disc space *(black arrow)* and epidural abscess *(white arrow).*

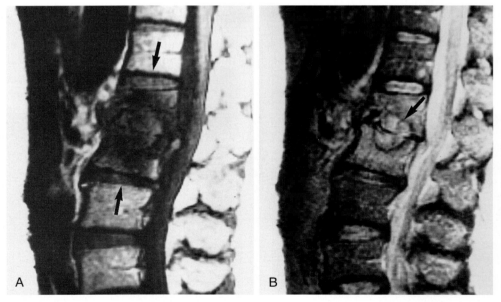

Figure 12–13. Osteomyelitis and spondylitis. Lumbar spine MRI of a woman with back pain. *(A)* On the sagittal T1WI, marrow signal intensity of the L2 and L3 vertebral bodies, which normally is bright, is dark *(arrows),* indicating replacement of marrow fat. The disc space is narrowed, and there is kyphosis at L2-L3. *(B)* On the sagittal T2WI, the marrow signal in the involved vertebral bodies is bright, and there is brighter fluid signal adjacent to the L2-L3 disc space *(arrow),* with partial disc destruction.

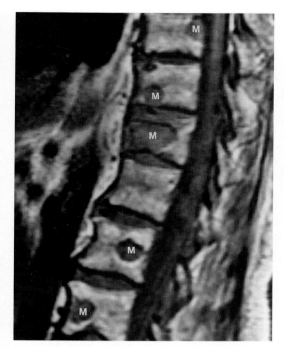

Figure 12–14. Marrow replacement in the spine from tumor. MRI (sagittal T1WI, no intravenous contrast administration) of a patient with myeloma. Multiple areas of lower signal intensity than normal fatty marrow represent replacement by tumor (M).

tion, in the absence of discitis. Clinically, patients with epidural abscess present with back pain and progressive neurologic deficits. Fever or leukocytosis may or may not be present. Because neurologic deterioration may occur over a period of hours, this lesion represents a surgical emergency. Unfortunately, the diagnosis can be missed on first presentation and appropriate imaging studies not obtained.

With an epidural abscess, the typical appearance of an extradural mass is observed on MRI, CT, or myelography. Compression of the thecal sac is frequently observed. Myelography should be performed only with great caution if epidural infection is suspected because there is a risk of seeding the cerebrospinal fluid (CSF). Neurologic deterioration resulting from acute decompression is another potential complication of myelography. MRI is particularly advantageous because it is noninvasive and very sensitive.

Marked enhancement with gadolinium is usually present (Fig. 12–15). Furthermore, adjacent soft tissues, which may be involved, are well visualized.

Arachnoiditis

Inflammation within the thecal sac from a variety of causes can lead to arachnoiditis. Etiologies include previous trauma, hemorrhage, surgery, and myelography with previously employed contrast agents. Clinical symptoms are varied but include neurologic deficit, diffuse back and lower extremity pain, and bowel and bladder symptoms. The nerve roots appear clumped together instead of spread evenly throughout the thecal sac. This may be observed on MRI, myelography, or postmyelography CT (Fig. 12–16). Severe arachnoiditis leads to a smooth or featureless thecal sac appearance on myelography, in which the nerve root sleeves are effaced and individual nerves are not distinguishable. Fibrotic masses can also occur within the thecal sac.

Meningitis

Meningitis can cause leptomeningeal MRI enhancement in the spine as well as around the brain. Uncomplicated meningitis is not an indication for spinal MRI, but occasionally contrasted MRI performed for complications of meningitis may disclose enhancement along the surface of the spinal cord. Tuberculosis and fungal infections may lead to chronic meningitis (Fig. 12–17). Abscess of the spinal cord itself is rare and has the imaging appearance of an intramedullary fluid-filled mass.

Arthritis

There are significant differences in the regional distribution of the various arthritides. The term *arthritis* is most properly applied to inflammatory joint diseases, many of which affect the spine. The sequelae of so-called osteoarthritic changes in the spine, which are not inflammatory in etiology, are discussed in the section on degenerative changes.

Rheumatoid arthritis (RA), known espe-

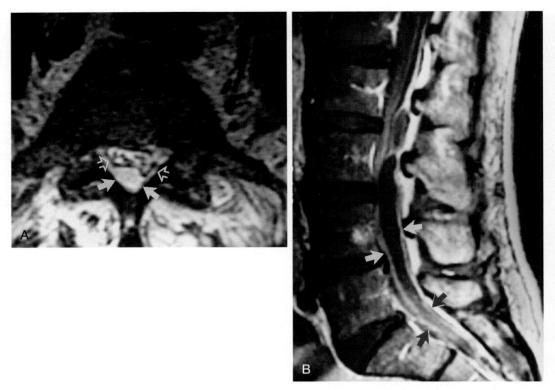

Figure 12–15. Spinal epidural abscess (without spondylitis). MRI of a man with gradual onset of lower extremity numbness and weakness. *(A)* Axial T2WI shows anterior displacement of the thecal sac (containing bright CSF and dark nerve roots, *open arrows*) by an epidural mass *(solid arrows)*. Fluid is also present in the paraspinous soft tissues. *(B)* Sagittal gadolinium-enhanced T1WI shows a rim-enhancing mass *(arrows)* with central low signal intensity of fluid filling much of the distal spinal canal. *S. aureus* epidural abscess was found at surgery.

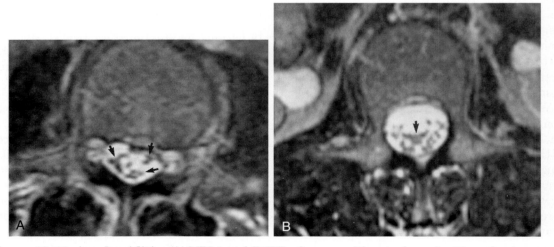

Figure 12–16. Arachnoiditis. *(A)* MRI (axial T2WI) of a man with spinal meningitis and prior surgery. The nerve roots of the cauda equina are clumped in an irregular manner *(arrows)*. *(B)* Axial T2WI of a different patient shows the normal appearance of nerve roots spread evenly through the posterior CSF space. The tip of the conus medullaris lies in the center *(arrow)*.

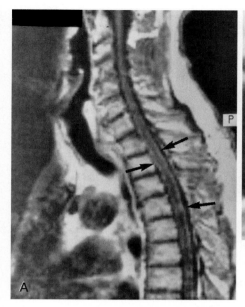
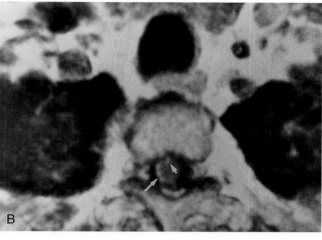

Figure 12–17. Tuberculous meningitis of the spine. MRI was performed on a former miner with silicosis and lower extremity weakness. *(A)* Sagittal and *(B)* axial post-gadolinium T1WI of the spine demonstrate thick, nodular areas of contrast enhancement along the surface of the spinal cord *(arrows).* Biopsy of this material revealed caseating granulomata.

cially for wrist and hand involvement, affects many joints throughout the body. The apophyseal (facet) joints of the spine are often involved. This can cause spondylolisthesis. In addition, the dens may be involved. Both the anterior and posterior synovial joints surrounding the dens may be affected (between the dens and anterior arch of C1 and between the dens and transverse ligament). Pannus (a reactive inflammatory mass) formation in RA may not only erode the dens, but can weaken the transverse ligament (Fig. 12–18). Atlantoaxial instability may ensue.

Plain films can reveal the bony changes of RA, but MRI is desirable to visualize the relationship of the dens or adjacent pannus to the spinal cord. Lateral flexion-extension views, with plain films or MRI, can assess the integrity of the transverse ligament. Atlantoaxial fusion may be necessary if the transverse ligament is not intact. Much less commonly, psoriatic or other arthritides can cause similar changes.

Ankylosis (immobility and fusion) of the spine is very common in ankylosing spondy-

litis. Acute or chronic trauma can lead to pseudoarthrosis (a false joint caused by pathologic fracture), most often at a single level. Severe degenerative change may then take place at that level.

NEOPLASMS AND OTHER MASSES OF THE SPINE

Intramedullary Neoplasms

Astrocytomas and ependymomas are the most common intramedullary tumors. These glial tumors expand the spinal cord. The imaging appearance reflects this anatomic alteration. Myelography or postmyelogram CT films demonstrate an enlarged spinal cord. However, MRI demonstrates much more soft tissue detail and is therefore the test of choice for intramedullary spinal cord tumors (Fig. 12–19). These neoplasms usually show increased signal intensity on T2-weighted images. Most spinal cord tumors are associated with some degree of enhancement following gadolinium administration.

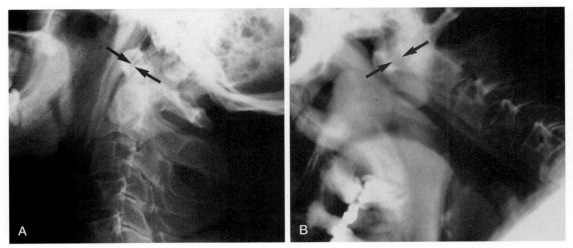

Figure 12–18. Transverse ligament damage from rheumatoid arthritis. *(A)* Lateral cervical spine radiograph in neutral position shows a normal relationship between the anterior arch of C1 and the odontoid process *(arrows)*. The odontoid process is smaller than normal because of erosion. *(B)* Lateral view in flexion demonstrates abnormal widening of the space between the anterior arch of C1 and the odontoid process *(arrows)*. There is a synovial space between the odontoid process and the transverse atlantal ligament. The ligament, which maintains the atlantodental relationship (normally less than or equal to 3 mm in adults), has been weakened by synovial inflammation.

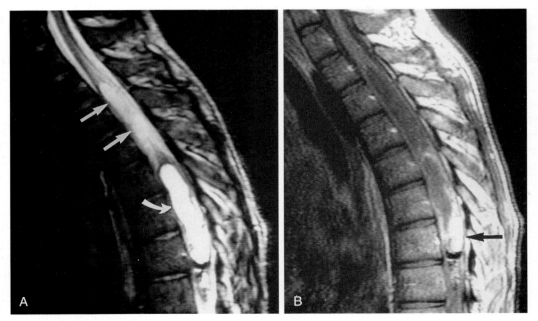

Figure 12–19. Intramedullary neoplasm. Thoracic spine MRI of a young man with myelopathy. *(A)* Sagittal T2WI reveals a large intramedullary mass *(straight arrows)* that expands the spinal cord. The astrocytoma contains a large cystic component *(curved arrow)*, and there is edema both rostral and caudal to the tumor. *(B)* After gadolinium administration (T1WI), enhancement is present in a portion of the tumor *(arrow)*.

Ependymoma of the spinal cord occurs most frequently in the cervical region in middle age. Ependymoma is the most common intramedullary tumor in adults. Pain is a typical presenting complaint. Neurologic deficits may also occur. Cysts and hemorrhage are common. Contrast enhancement is usually present, although it may be inhomogeneous.

Two histologic subtypes of ependymoma exist in the spine. The cellular subtype occurs primarily in the spinal cord, and the myxopapillary subtype occurs only in the conus medullaris region. The mean age of patients presenting with tumors in the conus medullaris and filum terminale (third decade) is lower than that in intramedullary ependymoma (fifth decade).

Astrocytoma is the most common spinal cord tumor in children. Most astrocytomas are low-grade tumors. Cervical and thoracic locations are most common, and pain is the most frequent initial complaint. The tumors frequently extend over multiple spinal segments. Cysts are common, and most astrocytomas enhance with gadolinium administration (see Fig. 12–19).

Hemangioblastomas are unusual spinal cord tumors. As in the brain, these are highly vascular and often have a large associated benign cyst with an enhancing nodule. Thoracic and cervical locations are most common. Approximately one-third of patients with spinal hemangioblastomas have von Hippel-Lindau disease (see Chapter 9).

Other Intramedullary Masses

Other causes of intramedullary masses also exist. Intramedullary metastases are uncommon. A syrinx is a relatively common cause of an expanded spinal cord. Hematoma, multiple sclerosis plaques, and transverse myelitis should also be considered as possible causes of spinal cord expansion and/or enhancement.

Intradural Extramedullary Neoplasms

The most common intradural extramedullary neoplasms are meningiomas and nerve sheath tumors. Nerve sheath tumors, including schwannomas and neurofibromas, are the most common of this group. The former are eccentric to the nerve, whereas the latter encase and are not separate from the nerve. However, because there is no reliable way to distinguish them by imaging, they are discussed together herein.

Plain films often demonstrate eroded pedicles and an enlarged neural foramen. A typical myelographic pattern consists of a mass within the thecal sac that is deviating the spinal cord. MRI signal intensity is variable (Fig. 12–20). Most nerve sheath tumors show contrast enhancement. Lesions that extend into a neural foramen often have a dumbbell-shaped appearance (Fig. 12–20*B*). Multiple nerve sheath tumors (see Fig. 9–22) should suggest the diagnosis of neurofibromatosis (see Chapter 9).

Patients with spinal meningiomas usually present in middle age. There is a greater female predominance of meningiomas in the spine (about 80%) than around the brain. The thoracic spine is the most common location. Calcification is rarely observed with spinal meningiomas. They usually appear as intradural masses that deviate the cord. The MRI appearance is similar to that of intracranial meningiomas. They are usually isointense with the spinal cord and demonstrate homogeneous gadolinium enhancement.

Subarachnoid spread of neoplasm is another cause of an intradural extramedullary mass. Medulloblastoma, ependymoma, astrocytoma, choroid plexus papilloma, and germinoma are all well known for subarachnoid spread. In addition to these central nervous system (CNS) tumors, breast and lung cancer, other solid tumors, and leukemia are also associated with leptomeningeal spread (Fig. 12–21). Evaluation of the spine for "drop" metastases is part of the staging evaluation for CNS tumors prone to such spread, especially medulloblastoma. MRI is the best test, and contrast material administration is mandatory. The imaging appearance includes multiple enhancing nodules along the surface of the spinal cord or nerve roots, and larger masses or sheets of tumor within the spinal canal.

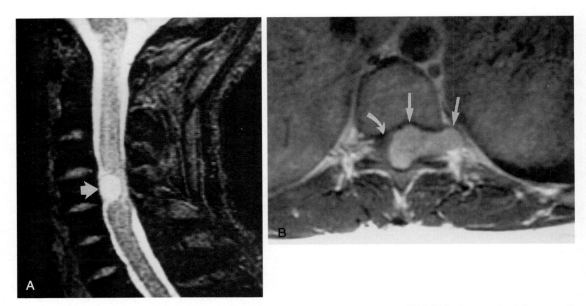

Figure 12–20. Intradural extramedullary nerve sheath tumors. *(A)* MRI of a man with neurofibromatosis (sagittal T2WI) shows a large oval mass *(arrow)* with higher signal intensity than the spinal cord. The spinal cord is severely compressed. *(B)* Axial post-gadolinium T1WI in a teenage girl demonstrates a dumbbell-shaped schwannoma *(straight arrows)* that deviates the spinal cord *(curved arrow)* to the right and extends into the left neural foramen.

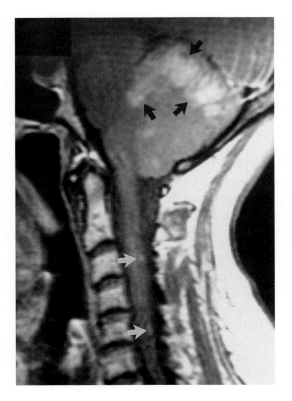

Figure 12–21. Meningeal carcinomatosis. MRI of a woman with a history of breast cancer. Sagittal post-gadolinium T1WI of the cervical spine shows extensive enhancement around the cerebellar folia *(black arrows),* and nodular enhancement along the surface of the medulla and cervical spinal cord *(white arrows).*

Other intradural extramedullary masses include lipomas (see Chapter 10), dermoid and epidermoid tumors, and arachnoid cysts.

Extradural Processes

Extradural masses most often originate in the bone. As they expand, they can impinge on the thecal sac and spinal cord. Metastatic disease is a common cause of an extradural neoplastic mass that can cause neurologic damage. Primary bone neoplasms, both benign and malignant, can also impinge on the neural foramina or spinal canal. The extradural origin is usually obvious on MRI or other tests (Fig. 12–22).

Radiation therapy is another cause of altered signal intensity of the marrow spaces. Edema may occur initially after radiation

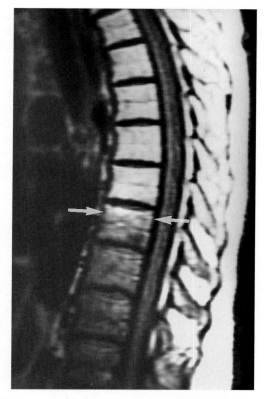

Figure 12–23. Fatty marrow after radiation. Sagittal MRI (T1WI) of a man who previously received radiation therapy for lung cancer. The very bright appearance of the marrow of the thoracic spine *(above arrows)* is the result of fatty replacement of normal cellular elements of marrow. The linear abrupt margin between normal and altered marrow *(arrows)* marks the edge of the radiation port.

therapy but is followed within a few weeks by increasing fat content of the marrow. This radiation change within bone is most often identified on T1-weighted MRI as high signal intensity in a well-circumscribed distribution corresponding to a radiation port (Fig. 12–23).

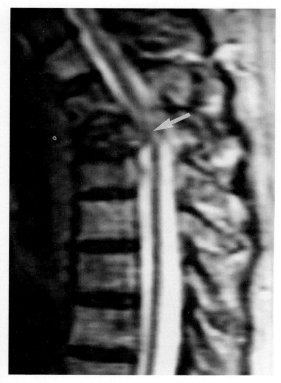

Figure 12–22. Spinal cord compression from vertebral tumor. MRI (sagittal T2WI) of an elderly man with prostate carcinoma and new myelopathy. Pathologic fracture of an upper thoracic vertebral body compresses the thoracic spinal cord *(arrow).* Signal intensity of the bone marrow is diffusely abnormal.

VASCULAR DISEASES OF THE SPINE

Vascular Malformations

Vascular malformations can affect the spine as well as the brain. The appearance on

MRI of cavernous malformations in the spine is similar to that in the brain. Typically, a reticulated area of blood products of varying ages with surrounding hemosiderin is observed.

Several types of spinal arteriovenous malformation (AVM) have been described, each with distinctive features. Intramedullary AVMs involve a nidus of abnormal vessels within the spinal cord. Enlarged feeding arteries and draining veins are also present (Fig. 12–24). Patients present most commonly in childhood or adolescence with subarachnoid hemorrhage or a spinal cord syndrome.

A perimedullary arteriovenous fistula (AVF) is a direct connection between an artery and vein on the surface of the spinal cord. Neurologic symptoms may be caused by venous hypertension.

A fistula can also occur within the dura mater. These dural AVFs are acquired and

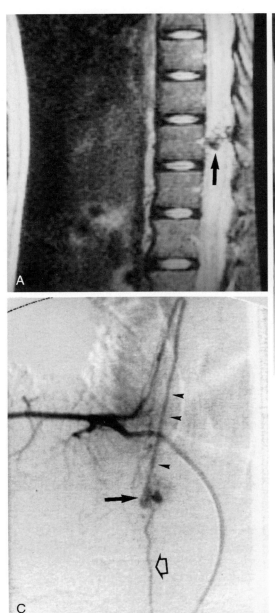

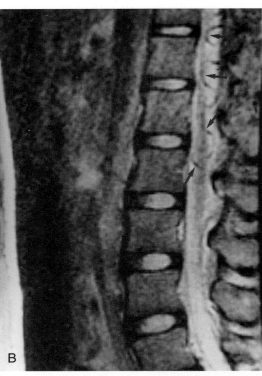

Figure 12–24. Spinal intramedullary AVM. MRI of a young woman with sudden onset of lower extremity weakness. *(A)* Sagittal T2WI at the thoracolumbar junction shows low signal intensity *(arrow)* within the spinal cord from acute hemorrhage. *(B)* Sagittal T2WI of the lumbar spine also reveals tortuous blood vessels (draining veins of the AVM, *arrows*). Arteriogram confirmed the presence of an intramedullary AVM with multiple feeding arteries. *(C)* AP view of digital subtraction arteriogram (injection of a right radiculomedullary artery) shows a feeding artery *(arrowheads)*, nidus *(solid arrow)*, and draining vein *(open arrow)*.

are observed most commonly in older men. Characteristic progressive myelopathy is again most likely the result of venous hypertension.

Diagnosis of these malformations can be quite difficult. MRI and MRA results may occasionally suggest the diagnosis. Hemorrhage within the spinal cord on MRI or evidence of ischemia can provide clues regarding the diagnosis of AVM. Myelography may demonstrate tortuous blood vessels on the surface of the spinal cord. Ultimately, the diagnosis of a spinal AVM or AVF rests with arteriography. It may be necessary to selectively catheterize multiple arteries to fully characterize a spinal malformation. In some cases, embolization may play a role in treatment.

Spinal Cord Ischemia

Spinal cord ischemia may result from trauma, atherosclerotic disease and other causes of emboli, and AVM. MRI is the most sensitive imaging tool for detecting suspected spinal cord ischemia. High signal intensity on T2-weighted MRI is observed with acute ischemia. However, increased signal alone is nonspecific, and, therefore, clinical correlation is mandatory.

DEMYELINATING DISEASE

Multiple Sclerosis

Multiple sclerosis (MS) frequently affects the spinal cord, and disability in patients with MS is often the result of spinal cord plaques. Plaques can occur anywhere, but the dorsal spinal cord is a common location (Fig. 12–25). MRI may demonstrate increased signal intensity (plaques) on T2-weighted sequences. As in the brain, areas of acute inflammation are often associated

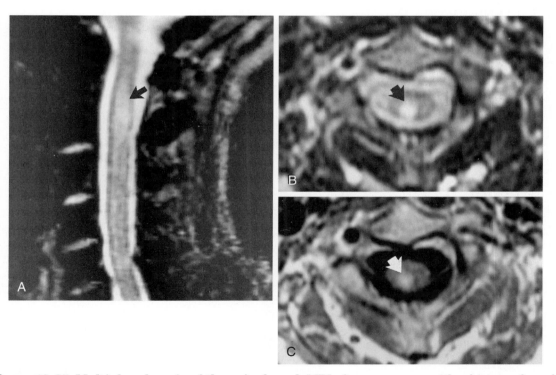

Figure 12–25. Multiple sclerosis of the spinal cord. MRI of young woman with a history of numbness that began in the right hand and progressed to involve the right upper extremity, trunk, and leg. *(A)* On the sagittal T2WI, an elongated region of increased signal intensity is present within the upper cervical spinal cord *(arrow)*. *(B)* On axial T2WI, the dorsolateral location of the plaque is demonstrated *(arrow)*. *(C)* After gadolinium administration (T2WI), there is contrast enhancement of the plaque *(arrow)*.

with contrast enhancement. The spinal cord may be swollen in the acute inflammatory stage. Myelomalacia may ensue with time.

Devic's Disease

Devic's disease is a form of demyelinating disease consisting of cervical spinal cord inflammation and necrosis as well as optic neuritis. MRI is the most sensitive imaging technique.

Transverse Myelitis

Transverse myelitis refers to acute inflammation of the spinal cord. It has been attributed to various causes, including infection, prior vaccination, and autoimmune disorders. A region of increased signal intensity is often observed on T2-weighted images of the spine. Contrast enhancement may be present (Fig. 12–26). The MRI appearance

of transverse myelitis and multiple sclerosis in the acute stage can be indistinguishable from that of an intramedullary neoplasm. Clinical findings must be sought to help separate these entities, because biopsy is undesirable for histologically benign diseases that may resolve on their own. Cranial MRI can sometimes provide supporting evidence for MS. In some cases, follow-up scans may be helpful.

SYRINX

Hydromyelia refers to a dilated central canal with an intact ependymal lining. *Syringomyelia* refers to a fluid space within the spinal cord that is not lined by ependyma. This histologic differentiation cannot be discerned on the basis of MRI or CT. Therefore, the less specific terms *syringohydromyelia*

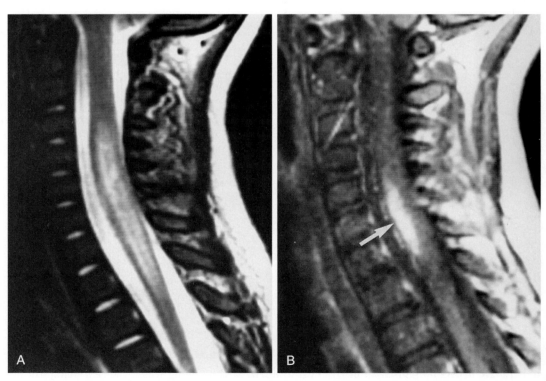

Figure 12–26. Transverse myelitis. Sagittal MRI of a child who developed a myelopathy after a viral infection. *(A)* On T2WI, the spinal cord is expanded, with central high signal intensity. *(B)* After gadolinium administration (T1WI), there is enhancement *(arrow)* within part of the area of signal abnormality. Six weeks later, the child's condition had improved markedly, and a repeat MRI was normal. Differential diagnosis of this MRI appearance on the initial scan includes tumor and MS.

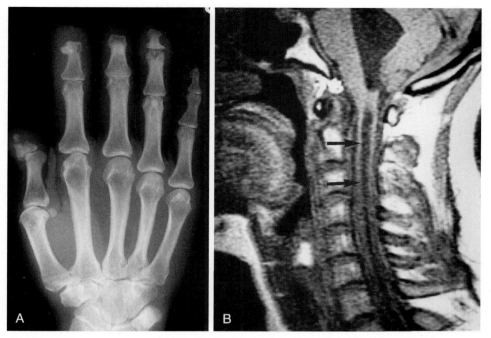

Figure 12–27. Syrinx. *(A)* AP radiograph of the right hand in this middle-aged woman with minimal pain sensation in the hands and a history of painless childbirth shows severe resorption of the distal phalanges. *(B)* MRI of the cervical spine (sagittal T1WI) reveals a large syrinx. Low signal intensity *(arrows)* is visible within the spinal cord.

or *syrinx* are often used. The imaging appearance is that of a fluid space within the spinal cord. MRI is the best test for imaging a syrinx (Fig. 12–27). A syrinx may be asymptomatic. However, dissociated sensory loss, a capelike distribution of sensory loss, weakness and atrophy because of anterior horn cell involvement, corticospinal weakness, and Horner's syndrome are frequent clinical findings.

Associated conditions include congenital anomalies, trauma, and neoplasms. Both Chiari I and Chiari II malformations are associated with syrinx (see Chapter 9, Fig. 9–2). With trauma, microcystic changes may coalesce and lead to a syrinx. Fluid spaces in or around a spinal cord neoplasm can represent either degeneration (necrosis) or syrinx. The former is usually contained within the tumor, and the latter usually lies either rostral or caudal to the tumor. (Note that the cysts that occur with many cases of hemangioblastoma are not themselves neoplastic. The tumor itself is a vascular nodule located in the wall of the cyst.) CT performed several hours after myelography may demonstrate the delayed appearance of contrast material within a syrinx and may occasionally help to distinguish a syrinx cavity from a tumor-associated cyst. However, MRI remains the best initial imaging test for intramedullary disease.

Further Readings

Chapter 1

Daniels DL, Haughton VM, Naidich TP. Cranial and Spinal Magnetic Resonance Imaging: An Atlas and Guide. Raven Press, New York, 1987.

Truwit CL, Lempert TE. High Resolution Atlas of Cranial Neuroanatomy. Williams & Wilkins, Baltimore, 1994.

Hayman LA, Hinck VC. Clinical Brain Imaging: Normal Structure and Functional Anatomy. Mosby–YearBook, St. Louis, 1992.

Orrison WW Jr, Lewine JD, Sanders JA, Hartshorne MF. Functional Brain Imaging. Mosby–YearBook, St. Louis, 1995.

Elster AD. Questions and Answers in Magnetic Resonance Imaging. Mosby–YearBook, St. Louis, 1994.

Newhouse JH, Wiener JI. Understanding MRI. Little, Brown, Boston, 1991.

Chapters 2–8

Osborn AG. Diagnostic Neuroradiology. Mosby–Year Book, St. Louis, 1994.

Atlas SW (ed). Magnetic Resonance Imaging of the Brain and Spine. Raven Press, New York, 1991.

Chapters 5 and 6

Osborn AG. Introduction to Cerebral Angiography. Harper & Row, Philadelphia, 1980.

Chapter 8

Tien RD, Felsberg GJ, Ferris NJ, Osumi AK. The dementias: Correlation of clinical features, pathophysiology, and neuroradiology. American Journal of Roentgenology 161:245–255, 1993.

Chapter 9

Barkovich AJ. Pediatric Neuroimaging (2nd edition). Raven Press, New York, 1995.

Wolpert SM, Barnes PD. MRI in Pediatric Neuroradiology. Mosby–YearBook, St. Louis, 1992.

Chapter 10

Barkovich AJ. Pediatric Neuroimaging (2nd edition). Raven Press, New York, 1995.

Osborne AG. Diagnostic Neuroradiology. Mosby–YearBook, St. Louis, 1994.

Chapter 11

Harris JH Jr, Mirvis SE. The Radiology of Acute Cervical Spine Trauma (3rd edition). Williams & Wilkins, Baltimore, 1995.

Hart BL, Orrison WW, Jr, Benzel EC. Imaging spine trauma. Spine: State of the Art Reviews 9:93–118. Hanley & Belfus, Philadelphia, 1995.

Chapter 12

Manelfe C (ed). Imaging of the Spine and Spinal Cord. Raven Press, New York, 1992.

Enzmann DR, DeLaPaz RL, Rubin JB. Magnetic Resonance of the Spine. Mosby, St. Louis, 1990.

Modic MT, Masaryk J, Ross JS. Magnetic Resonance Imaging of the Spine (2nd edition). Mosby, St. Louis, 1994.

Appendix 1

Sizes of Extra-Axial Hematomas

The following examples are provided to facilitate communication about the size of extra-axial hematomas. A single image provides limited information, and the number of CT slices upon which the hematoma was visible is indicated for each of the following cases. Volume estimates in the following examples are based on volumetric measurements of multiple slices and, when available, from surgical information.

Size is only one of several important elements to consider in assessing the significance of such hematomas. Evidence of mass effect may be manifested by effacement of underlying sulci, deformity of the ventricles or subarachnoid cisterns, or midline shift. Other injuries such as contusions, shearing injury, or edema of the brain may be more important than extra-axial blood collections. Pre-existing atrophy may lessen the effect of subdural or epidural hematomas. These factors are discussed in Chapter 2. Moreover, imaging studies are important but cannot be judged in isolation; clinical condition of the patient remains the central consideration in management decisions. In other words, treat the patient, not the scan!

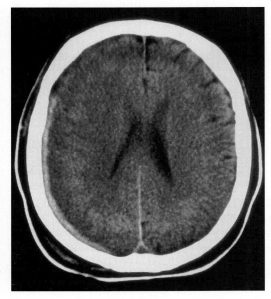

S1. Small subdural hematoma (approximately 20 ml). Hematoma visible on seven slices of 10 mm thickness. There is a typical crescentic configuration.

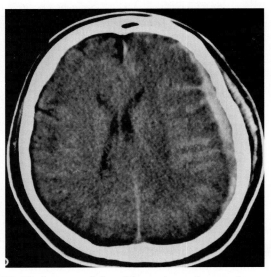

S2. Moderate subdural hematoma (approximately 40–50 ml). Hematoma visible on nine 10-mm-thick slices. There is a midline shift.

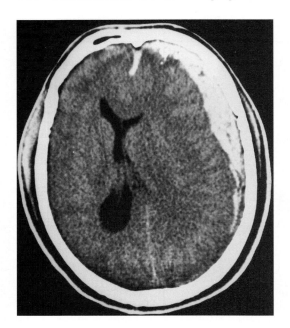

S3. Very large subdural hematoma (approximately 85–105 ml). Hematoma visible on 15 5-mm-thick slices and three 10-mm-thick slices. Severe mass effect. See Figure 2–11 for illustration of other levels from the same case and evidence of uncal herniation.

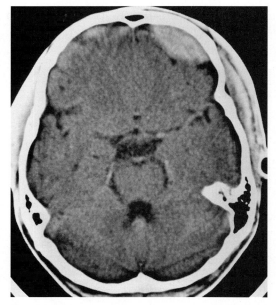

E1. Small epidural hematoma (approximately 10 ml). Hematoma visible on eight 5-mm-thick slices. There is a typical biconvex configuration.

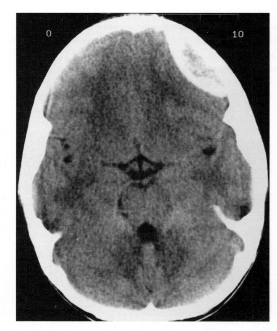

E2. Moderate epidural hematoma (approximately 30–40 ml). Hematoma visible on six 5-mm-thick slices and three 10-mm-thick slices (same case as Fig. 2–2). The epidural hematoma in Figure 2–3 has essentially the same volume. Despite the similar size of the hematomas, the clinical course of the two patients was quite different because of significant associated brain injury in the second case.

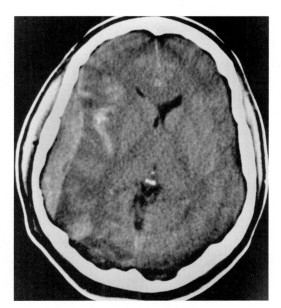

E3. Large epidural hematoma (approximately 60–75 ml). Hematoma visible on six 5-mm-thick slices and four 10-mm-thick slices. The configuration, elongated and crescentic on some slices, is somewhat unusual for an epidural hematoma. Subdural versus epidural location of an extra-axial hematoma cannot always be determined accurately on CT. Epidural location of the hematoma, subarachnoid hemorrhage, and contusion of the underlying brain were all confirmed surgically in this case.

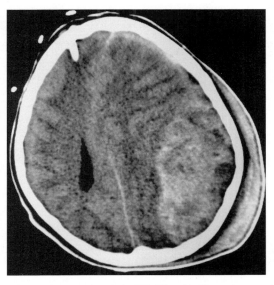

E4. Very large epidural hematoma (approximately 75–90 ml). Hematoma visible on nine 5-mm-thick slices.

Appendix 2

Approach to Imaging of Common Diagnostic Problems

The following is an approach to the initial imaging of common CNS problems. Such imaging studies are usually satisfactory and appropriate; but, these are suggestions only. Extensive scientific data are lacking regarding the optimal diagnostic tests for many indications. Numerous factors enter into the decision about CNS imaging studies, including patient history, patient compliance, local availability of technology, cost, and individual experience of both the ordering and the interpreting physicians.

Indication for Imaging	Imaging Studies
Head injury, acute	CT without contrast (see Chapter 2)
Head injury, follow-up or late imaging	MRI without contrast (see Chapter 2)
Head injury, possible child abuse	CT without contrast and skull films (part of skeletal survey; MRI in selected cases, see Chapter 9)
Infection, suspected meningitis	CT without contrast (see Chapter 3)
Infection, possible abscess	CT with contrast or MRI with contrast (see Chapter 3)
Infection, immunocompromised patient	MRI without contrast; MRI with contrast if meningeal or ependymal processes suspected or to further evaluate parenchymal disease (see Chapter 3)
Stroke, acute	CT without contrast (to exclude hemorrhage, see Chapter 5)
Seizures, new onset in a child	MRI (best for congenital malformations, see Chapter 9)
Seizures, new onset in an adult	MRI without contrast or CT with contrast (MRI more sensitive for many processes)
Seizures, partial complex or temporal lobe origin	MRI without contrast, including coronal plane imaging for evaluation of the hippocampus (see Chapter 9)

Suspected multiple sclerosis	MRI without contrast (see Chapter 8)
Dementia	MRI without contrast (see Chapter 8)
Pituitary dysfunction	MRI, thin sections through sella turcica, without and with contrast
Suspected acoustic schwannoma	MRI of internal auditory canal region, with contrast or high-resolution T2-weighted series without contrast
Low back pain	No imaging for 6 to 8 weeks or more of conservative therapy unless major neurologic deficits or other complications; MRI or CT without contrast; MRI preferred by many surgeons for preoperative planning, and MRI is more sensitive for a variety of spine processes (see Chapter 12)
Neck pain	Plain films, MRI; as with low back pain, imaging should be done only after consideration of clinical factors and after a trial of conservative therapy (see Chapter 12)
Neurogenic claudication	MRI without contrast or CT without contrast (see Chapter 12)
Myelopathy	MRI; consider contrast for possible neoplasm
Cervical spine trauma, acute	Plain films; CT without contrast for additional evaluation of possible fractures; MRI without contrast for evaluation of spinal cord injury or for possible major acute ligamentous injury (see Chapter 11)

Index

Note: Page numbers in *italic* refer to illustrations;
page numbers followed by t refer to tables.

A

Abscess, epidural, 169–171, *172*
  pyogenic, 27t, 27–28, *29*
Abuse, child, brain injury in, 130,
  131
ACA (anterior cerebral artery), *70*,
  70–72, *71*
Acoustic schwannoma, 60, *60*
Acquired immunodeficiency
  syndrome (AIDS), 33, *33*
  lymphoma in, *48*
  perinatal, 37
  toxoplasmosis in, 34, *35*
  tuberculous meningitis in, 28, *30*
Acute disseminated encephalomyelitis (ADEM), 31–33
  in white matter disease, 105
Adenoma, pituitary, *56*, 56–57, *57*
Adrenoleukodystrophy (ALD), 107,
  107
Agenesis, of corpus callosum, *114*,
  114–115
Aging, in degenerative diseases,
  108, *108*
Agyria, 119
AIDS (acquired immunodeficiency
  syndrome), 33, *33*
  lymphoma in, *48*
  perinatal, 37
  toxoplasmosis in, 34, *35*

AIDS (acquired immunodeficiency
  syndrome) *(Continued)*
  tuberculous meningitis in, 28, *30*
Air, characteristics of, on CT, 2
  on MRI, 8, 8t
ALD (adrenoleukodystrophy), 107,
  107
Alexander's disease, 107
Alzheimer's disease, 109–110
Aneurysm(s), berry, 85–88, 86t
  cavernous sinus, 57, *59*
  dissecting, 88, *88*
  giant, 85
  intracranial, *81*, 85–88, 86t, *87*
  saccular, *81*, 86
Angiography. See also *Digital
  subtraction angiography
  (DSA)*.
  of arteriovenous malformations,
  89
  of carotid artery, 72–73, *73*
  of dissecting aneurysms, 88, *88*
  of intracranial aneurysms, *81*,
  86–87
  of spinal artery, *137*
  of vascular blush, 50, *55*
  of venous infarction, 75, *77*
Angioma, cavernous, 91, *92*
  venous, 91, *92*
Ankylosis, 173
Anterior cerebral artery (ACA), *70*,
  70–72, *71*

Apoplexy, pituitary, 57
Aqueductal obstruction, in
  hydrocephalus, 97–99, *99*, 99t
Arachnoid cyst, 117, *118*
Arachnoiditis, 171, *172*
Arnold-Chiari malformation,
  112–114, *113*
Arterial occlusion, 67–72
  arterial territories in, *70*, 70–72,
  71
  evolution of, *70*, 72
  imaging appearance of, 67–70,
  68–71
Arteriography, of arteriovenous
  malformations, *90*
  of dissecting aneurysms, 88, *88*
Arteriovenous fistula (AVF), 178
  dural, 89–91, *91*
Arteriovenous malformation
  (AVM), in brain, 88–91, 89t,
  90, *91*
  in spine, 177–179, *178*
Artery(ies), carotid. See *Carotid
  artery*.
  cerebellar, *71*, 72
  cerebral. See *Cerebral artery*.
  occlusion of. See *Arterial occlusion*.
  of Adamkiewicz, 135
  spinal, *137*
Arthritis, 171–173, *174*

Aspergillosis, in immunocompromised patient, 34
Astrocytoma(s), 40–43, *41–44*
  brainstem, 43, *44*
  cerebellar, 43, *44*
    of posterior fossa, 100
  in tuberous sclerosis, *126*
  intramedullary, 138t, 173–175
Atherosclerosis, carotid artery, 72–74, *73*
Atrophy, cerebellar, *109*, 110
  hydrocephalus versus, 95–96, *97*
Auditory canal, neuroma of, *60*, 60–63
AVF (arteriovenous fistula), 178
  dural, 89–91, *91*
AVM (arteriovenous malformation), in brain, 88–91, 89t, *90*, *91*
  in spine, 177–179, *178*
Avulsion, of spinous processes, 153, *155*
Axial loading injury, 150–152
Axonal injury, diffuse, 16

B

Back pain, 161
Bacterial meningitis, 25
Ball-valve effect, in hydrocephalus, 96–97
Basal ganglia, in focal brain damage, 76
  in hypoxic injury, 74, *75*
  in multiple sclerosis, 104
  on cross-sectional imaging, *3*
Basilar cisterns, CSF flow obstruction at, 100
Battered child syndrome, 130
Berry aneurysm, 85–88, 86t
Bitemporal hemianopsia, in pituitary adenomas, 57
Blood, appearance of, on MRI, 82, 83t
  characteristics of, on CT, 2
  on MRI, 8, 8t
  supply of, to spinal cord, 135, *137*
Bone, on MRI, 8, 8t
Border zone infarction, 74, *74*
Brain. See also *Cerebral; Cerebro-* entries.
  abscess of, 27t, 27–28, *29*
  congenital malformation(s) of, 111–119
    cephalocele as, 111–112, *112*
    Chiari malformation as, *112*, 112–114, *113*
    corpus callosum disorders in, 114–115, *114–116*
    cystic malformation as, 116–117, *117*, *118*
    holoprosencephalies as, 115, *116*

Brain *(Continued)*
    neuronal migration disorders in, 117–119, *119–122*
    septo-optic dysplasia in, 115–116, *117*
  degenerative disease(s) of, 103–110
    aging and, 108, *108*
    cerebellar atrophy as, *109*, 110
    dementia as, 108–110
    demyelinating diseases as, 107, *107*
    deposition diseases as, 108
    Huntington's disease as, 110
    movement disorders in, 108–110
    multiple sclerosis as, 103–105, *104–106*
    reversible changes of vascular origin in, *109*, 110
    white matter disease as, 105
  infection(s) of, 27–33
    cerebritis and pyogenic abscess as, 27t, 27–28, *29*
    encephalitis as, 28, *30*
    fungi as, 29, *31*
    parasites in, 29–31, *32*, 32t, *33*
    syphilis as, 31
    tuberculosis as, 28–29, *30*, *31*
    virus in, 31–33
  injury to, 15–18
    in child abuse, 130, *131*
    metabolic conditions resulting in, 76–78, *78*
  neoplasms of, 39–65
    classification of, 39–40
    evaluation of, 39, 40t
    metastases of, 51–56, *55*. See also *Metastasis(es)*.
    of cerebellopontine angle, *60*, 60t, 60–63
    of glial-cell origin, 40–45. See also *Glioma(s)*.
    of meninges, 49–51, *54*, *55*
    of non–glial-cell origin, 45–49. See also *Non–glial-cell tumor(s)*.
    of sellar region, 56–59, 56–60, 60t
    treatment of, *61*, 63–64
  on cross-sectional imaging, 1–2, *3–6*
  radiation injury to, *61*, 63–64
  vascular diseases of, 67–78. See also *Ischemia*.
Brain death, 74–75, *76*
Brainstem, astrocytoma of, 43, *44*
  glioma of, 100
  on cross-sectional imaging, *6*
Breast carcinoma, metastasis of, 51–52
Burst fracture(s), of cervical spine, *152*, 152–153

Burst fracture(s) *(Continued)*
  of thoracic and lumbar spine, 157, *158*
Butterfly glioma, 42, *42*

C

Calcification, in Sturge-Weber syndrome, *128*
Canalization, 137
  abnormal, *139*, *141*, 142–143
Canavan's disease, 107, *107*
Capillary telangiectasia, 91–92
Carcinoma, metastasis of, 51–52
Carcinomatosis, meningeal, 175, *176*
Carotid artery, 70, 70–72, *71*
  atherosclerosis of, 72–74, *73*
  cavernous sinus aneurysm in, 57, *59*
  occlusion of, 67, *68*, *69*
  traumatic dissection of, 88, *88*
Carotid-cavernous fistula, 92–93, *93*
Caudal regression, *141*, 142–143
Cavernous angioma, 91, *92*
Cavernous sinus aneurysm, 57, *59*
Central nervous system, infection of, 25–37. See also *Infection*.
Central pontine myelinolysis, 77
Cephalocele, 111–112, *112*
Cerebellar artery, *71*, 72
Cerebellar astrocytoma, 43, *44*
  of posterior fossa, 100
Cerebellar atrophy, *109*, 110
Cerebellar tonsil herniation, 18
Cerebellopontine angle (CPA), epidermoid tumor of, 48, *51*
  masses of, *60*, 60t, 60–63
Cerebral artery, anterior, 70, 70–72, *71*
  middle, 70, 70–72, *71*
    infarction of, 68, *69*
  posterior, *71*, 72
Cerebral atrophy, 95
Cerebral contusion, 16, *17*
Cerebral venous thrombosis, 77
Cerebritis, 27t, 27–28, *29*
Cerebrospinal fluid (CSF), characteristics of, on CT, 2
  on MRI, 8, 8t
  in neoplasm metastasis, 56
  in ventricles, 1–2
  leaks of, in skull fractures, 20–21
  obstruction of, 95, 96, *96*
Cervical herniated nucleus pulposus, *163*
Cervical trauma, 146–155
  burst fractures in, *152*, 152–153
  cautions for, 155
  cervicocranial disruption in, 150
  C1 fractures in, *150*, 150–151

Cervical trauma *(Continued)*
  C2 fractures in, *151,* 151–152,
    152
  evaluation of, 146–149, *146–149*
  extension injuries in, 153–155
  flexion injuries in, 153, *154, 155*
  rotational injuries in, 153, *156*
Cervicocranial junction, dislocation
    at, 150
  imaging of, 146
Cervicothoracic junction,
    visualization of, 146, *146*
Chance fracture, 157, *158*
Chiari malformation(s), *112,*
    112–114, *113*
  in ventricular obstruction, 100,
    101
Child. See also *Infant.*
  brain injury in, 130, *131*
  cervical spine of, 149, *149*
  neuroradiology for, 111–133. See
    also *Pediatric neuroradiol-
    ogy.*
Choroid plexus papilloma, *46*
Choroid plexus tumor, 45, *46*
Choroidal fissure cyst, 117, *118*
Clay-shoveler's fracture, 153, *155*
Closed head injury, *15–18,* 16–18
CMV (cytomegalovirus), in
    immunocompromised patient,
    34
  perinatal, 35
Coccidioidomycosis meningitis, 29,
    31
Colloid cyst, 97, *98*
Communicating hydrocephalus,
    100–101
  in subarachnoid hemorrhage, 79
Compression fracture, of thoracic
    and lumbar spine, 157, *157*
Computed tomography (CT), of
    arterial occlusion, 67–70,
    68–71
  of astrocytoma, 40, *41,* 42–43,
    43, 44
  of basal ganglia, *3*
  of brain, postnatal acquired dis-
    orders of, 130–132, *131*
    radiation injuries and, 64
  of brain death, 76
  of brainstem, *6*
  of butterfly glioma, 42, *42*
  of Chiari malformation, *101*
  of colloid cyst, *98*
  of congenital infection, *36*
  of corpus callosum, *116*
  of cranial trauma, 11–24. See
    also *Cranial trauma.*
  of craniopharyngioma, 57, *58*
  of craniosynostosis, 133
  of cysticercosis, *33*
  of diastematomyelia, *142,* 143
  of global ischemia, *74*
  of herniated nucleus pulposus,
    162

Computed tomography (CT)
    (Continued)
  of internal capsule, *3*
  of intracranial aneurysm, 86–87,
    87
  of intracranial hemorrhage, 79–
    82, *81–84*
  of lipoma, *116*
  of lipomyelomeningocele, 140
  of medulloblastoma, *47*
  of mega cisterna magna, *117*
  of meningioma, 50
  of meningitis, *26*
  of metastases, 52
  of midbrain, *4*
  of multiple sclerosis, 104–105,
    105
  of oligodendroglioma, *45*
  of pons, *5*
  of posterior longitudinal liga-
    ment, *167*
  of schizencephaly, *120*
  of spine, 135–137, *136, 137,*
    138t, *139*
    trauma to, 145
  of Sturge-Weber syndrome, *128*
  of subarachnoid hemorrhage, 86
  of systemic lupus erythemato-
    sus, *109*
  of tuberous sclerosis, *126*
  of venous infarction, 75–76, *77*
  of ventricle, *5*
  techniques of, 2
C1 fracture, *150,* 150–151
Congenital infection(s), 35–37, *36,*
    37t
Congenital malformation(s), of
    brain, 111–119. See also
    *Brain, congenital malforma-
    tion(s) of.*
  of posterior fossa, 100
  of spine, 137–143. See also
    Spine.
Congenital rubella, *36,* 37
Conjoined nerve root(s), 164, *165*
Contrast agent(s), in CT, 2
  in MRI, 8–9
Contrecoup injury, 16
Contusion(s), *15–17,* 16
  in skull fractures, 20, *22*
Corpus callosum, disorders of,
    114–115, *114–116*
  in multiple sclerosis, 104
Cortical contusion, 16, *16*
  in skull fractures, 20, *22*
Coup injury, 16
CPA (cerebellopontine angle),
    epidermoid tumor of, 48, *51*
  masses of, *60,* 60t, 60–63
Cranial trauma, 11–24
  brain injury in, 15–18
  epidural hematomas in, 11–12,
    12, 13
  intracranial herniations in, 18,
    19, 20

Cranial trauma *(Continued)*
  intraventricular hemorrhage in,
    15
  late effects of, 24
  skull fractures in, *17,* 18–24, *21,
    22.* See also *Skull.*
  subarachnoid hemorrhage in, *12,*
    15, *15*
  subdural hematomas in, *12,* 13–
    14, *14, 15*
Craniopharyngioma, 57, *58*
Craniosynostosis, 132–133, *133*
Cranium. See *Skull.*
Cryptococcal meningitis, 34, *36*
Cryptococcosis, 34
CSF. See *Cerebrospinal fluid
    (CSF).*
C6-C7 subluxation, *146*
CT. See *Computed tomography
    (CT).*
C2 fracture, *151,* 151–152, *152*
Cut-film technique, in carotid
    artery evaluation, 73
Cystic malformation(s), 116–117,
    117, 118
Cysticercosis, 30–31, *32,* 32t, *33*
Cyst(s), arachnoid, 117, *118*
  choroidal fissure, 117, *118*
  colloid, 97, *98*
  dermoid, 49, *52*
    in failure of disjunction, 140–
      142, *141*
  epidermoid, 48, *51,* 64t
    in failure of disjunction, 140
  leptomeningeal, *23,* 24
  of von Hippel-Lindau syndrome,
    127
  Rathke's cleft, 57
Cytomegalovirus (CMV), in
    immunocompromised patient,
    34
  perinatal, 35

D

Dandy-Walker malformation, *115,*
    116–117, *117*
  in ventricular obstruction, 100
Dandy-Walker variant, 117, *117*
Death, brain, 74–75, *76*
Degenerative disease(s), of brain,
    103–110. See also *Brain.*
  of spine, 161–167. See also
    Spine.
Dementia, 108–110
Demyelinating disease(s), of brain,
    103–107, *104–107*
  of spinal cord, *179,* 179–180, *180*
Deposition disease(s), 108
Depressed skull fracture, 16, *17*
Dermal sinus, 140–142, *141*
Dermoid cyst, 140–142, *141*
Dermoid tumor(s), 49, *52*

Devic's disease, 180
Diastematomyelia, *142*, 143
Diffuse axonal injury, 16
Digital subtraction angiography
(DSA), of carotid artery, 72–73
of spinal artery, *137*
Disc, infection of, 167–169,
169–171
MRI evaluation of, 157
protrusion of, 162–164, *163–165*
Discitis, 167
Disjunction, failure of, 140–142,
141
premature, 140, *140*
Dislocation, at cervicocranial
junction, 150
of facet joints, 153, *155*, *156*
Dissecting aneurysm, 88, *88*
Dissection, carotid artery, 88, *88*
Disseminated encephalomyelitis,
31–33
in white matter disease, 105
Doppler ultrasound, in carotid
artery evaluation, 73
technique of, 9
Dorsal dermal sinus, 140–142, *141*
Drop metastasis, in intradural
extramedullary compartment,
136, 138t
DSA (digital subtraction
angiography), of carotid artery,
72–73
of spinal artery, *137*
Dural arteriovenous fistula, 89–91,
91
Dural sinus thrombosis, 75–76, *77*
Duret hemorrhage, 18, *20*
Dysplasia, septo-optic, 115–116,
117

E

Echo time (TE), 7
Edema, characteristics of, on CT, 2
on MRI, 8, 8t
Embolic infarction, 67
Empyema, epidural, 26–27
subdural, 26, *28*
Encephalitis, 28, *30*
Encephalocele, 111
Encephalomalacia, *70*
Encephalomyelitis, 31–33
in white matter disease, 105
Encephalopathy, hypertensive, 110
Encephalotrigeminal angiomatosis,
127
Ependymitis, 28
Ependymoma(s), 45, *45*
intramedullary, 138t, 173–175
posterior fossa, 100
Epidermoid tumor, 48, *51*
in failure of dysjunction, 140
radiographic features of, 64t

Epidural abscess, 169–171, *170*,
172
Epidural empyema, in meningitis,
26–27
Epidural hematoma, 11–12, *12*, *13*
in skull fractures, 20, *22*
Escobar classification, of
neurocysticercosis, 32t
Extension injury(ies), of cervical
spine, 153–155
Extra-axial empyema, in
meningitis, 26–27, *28*
Extra-axial hematoma, 11–14,
12–15
size of, 185, *185–187*
Extradural process(es), 137, 138t,
177, *177*
Extramedullary intradural
neoplasm, 175–177, *176*
Extramedullary intradural
process(es), 136, 138t, *139*
Extraventricular obstruction,
100–101

F

Facet joint, disruption of, 153, *155*,
156
Falx cerebri, herniation under, 18,
19
Fat, characteristics of, on CT, 2
on MRI, 7–8, 8t
Filum terminale, lipoma of, 140
Fistula, carotid-cavernous, 92–93,
93
dural arteriovenous, 89–91, *91*
Flexion injury(ies), of cervical
spine, 153, *154*, *155*
Flexion teardrop fracture, 153
Foramen of Monro, mass at, 96, *98*
Fracture(s), of cervical spine,
150–152, *150–152*
burst, *152*, 152–153
extension injuries in, 153–155
flexion injuries in, 153, *154*,
155
rotational injuries in, 153, *156*
of skull, 17, 18–24, *21*, *22*
CSF leaks in, 20–21
depressed, 16, *17*
growing, 21–24, *23*
temporal bone, 21, *23*
of thoracic and lumbar spine,
155–157, *157*, *158*
Fungal infection, 29, *31*
in immunocompromised patient,
30, 34, *36*

G

Gadolinium, in MRI, 8–9

Ganglia, basal, in focal brain
damage, 76
in hypoxic injury, 74, *75*
in multiple sclerosis, 104
on cross-sectional imaging, 3
Ganglioglioma, 48, *50*
Germ-cell tumor, 48–49, *51–53*, 64t
Germinal matrix hemorrhage,
127t, 127–128
Germinoma, 49, *53*
Giant aneurysm, 85
Glioblastoma multiforme, 40,
41–42
Glioma(s), 40–45
astrocytoma as, 40–43, *41–44*
brainstem, 100
butterfly, 42, *42*
choroid plexus tumors as, 45, *46*
ependymoma as, 45, *45*
oligodendroglioma as, 43–45, *45*
optic, 57
Granulomatous infection, as
immunocompromised patient,
30, 34, *36*
Gray matter, characteristics of, on
CT, 2
on MRI, 8, 8t
heterotopic, 119, *119*
Growing skull fracture, 21–24, *23*
Gunshot wound, cranial, 15–16, *16*

H

Hangman's fracture, 152, *152*
Head trauma. See *Cranial trauma.*
Hemangioblastoma(s), 46–48, *49*
intramedullary, 138t
spinal cord, 175
Hemangioma, 64t
Hemangiopericytoma, 50–51
Hematogenous metastasis, 51–52,
55
Hematoma(s), epidural, 11–12, *12*,
13
in skull fractures, 20, *22*
sizes of, 185, *185–187*
subdural, *12*, 13–14, *14*, *15*
herniation in, 18, *19*, *20*
Hemianopsia, bitemporal, 57
Hemorrhage, Duret, 18, *20*
germinal matrix, 127t, 127–128
hypertensive, 93
in chronic infarction, 72
in pituitary adenomas, 57
intracranial, 79–94. See also *Intracranial hemorrhage.*
intraventricular, 15, 79–80, *81*,
129
lobar, 93
midbrain, 15, *15*
parenchymal, 80, *81*, 127–128,
130
subarachnoid, *12*, 15, *15*, 79, *81*

Hemorrhage *(Continued)*
    Hunt and Hess grading system of, 86t
    with intracranial aneurysms, 85–86
Herniation(s), intracranial, 18, *19, 20*
    of nucleus pulposus, 137, 162–164, *163–165*
    MRI evaluation of, 157
Herpes encephalitis, 28, *30*
Herpes simplex infection, perinatal, 37
Heterotopic gray matter, 119, *119*
Hippocampal sclerosis, 132, *132*
Histiocytosis, *64,* 64t, 65
HIV (human immunodeficiency virus) infection. See *Acquired immunodeficiency syndrome (AIDS).*
HNP (herniated nucleus pulposus), 137, 162–164, *163–165*
    MRI evaluation of, 157
Holoprosencephaly, 115, *116*
Human immunodeficiency virus (HIV) infection. See *Acquired immunodeficiency syndrome (AIDS).*
Hunt and Hess grading system, for subarachnoid hemorrhage, 85, 86t
Huntington's disease, 110
Hydrocephalus, 95–101
    atrophy versus, 95–96, *97*
    Chiari malformations and, *113,* 114
    communicating, 100–101
    in subarachnoid hemorrhage, 79
    in intracranial hemorrhage, 80
    in meningitis, 25, *26*
    normal pressure, 95–96, *97*
    obstruction in, *96,* 96–101
        aqueductal, 97–99, *99,* 99t
        congenital posterior fossa anomalies in, 100
        extraventricular, 100–101
        lateral ventricle, 96, 97t
        posterior fossa masses in, 99–100, 100t
        third ventricle, 96–97, *98*
    treatment of, imaging following, 101, *101*
    ultrasound of, *129*
Hydromyelia, 138t, 180
Hygroma, in meningitis, 25–26, *26, 27*
Hyperextension, of cervical spine, 153–155
Hypertension, encephalopathy in, 110
    hemorrhage in, 93
    intracranial hemorrhage from, 80, *81*

Hypoperfusion, in cerebral ischemia, 74, *74, 75*
Hypoxia, in cerebral ischemia, 74, *74, 75*

I

IAC (internal auditory canal), neuroma of, *60,* 60–63
ICA (internal carotid artery), 70, 70–72, *71*
    cavernous sinus aneurysm in, 57, *59*
    occlusion of, 67, *68, 69*
Imaging technique(s), 1–10
    brain anatomy in, 1–2, *3–6*
    for CT, 2
    for magnetic source imaging, 10
    for MRI, 6–9, 8t
    for nuclear medicine, 9–10
    for PET, 10
    for ultrasound, 9
Immunocompromised patient, infections in, 33–34, *33–36*
Inborn errors of metabolism, 107
Infant. See also *Child.*
    premature, evaluation of, 127t, 127–130, *129, 130*
Infarction, border zone, 74, *74*
    embolic, 67
    middle cerebral artery, 68, *69*
    posterior cerebral artery, *71,* 72
    posterior inferior cerebellar artery, *71,* 72
    thrombotic, in arterial occlusion, 67–70, *68–71*
    in venous occlusion, 75, *77*
    venous, 75–76, *77*
Infection, 25–37
    in immunocompromised patient, 33–34, *33–36*
    of brain, 27–33. See also *Brain infection(s) of.*
    of meninges, 25–27, *26–28*
    of spine, 167–173. See also *Spine, infection(s) of.*
    perinatal, 35–37, *36,* 37t
    intracranial, 132
Injury. See *Trauma;* and at specific site, e.g., *Spine, trauma to.*
Internal auditory canal (IAC), neuroma of, *60,* 60–63
Internal capsule, on cross-sectional imaging, *3*
Internal carotid artery (ICA), 70, 70–72, *71*
    cavernous sinus aneurysm of, 57, *59*
    occlusion of, 67, *68, 69*
Intersegmental laminar fusion, 143
Intervertebral disc, infection of, 167–169, *169–171*

Intervertebral disc *(Continued)*
    MRI evaluation of, 157
Intracranial aneurysm, *81,* 85–88, 86t, *87*
Intracranial hemorrhage, 79–94
    causes of, 80t
    CT appearance of, 80–82, *81–84*
    dissecting aneurysm in, 88, *88*
    hypertensive, 93
    intracranial aneurysm in, *81,* 85–88, 86t
    intraventricular, 79–80, *81*
    lobar, 93
    MRI appearance of, *82–84,* 82–85, 83t
    neoplasms in, 94, *94*
    parenchymal, 80, *81*
    perinatal, 127t, 127–128, *129*
    subarachnoid, 79, *81*
    vascular malformations in, 88–93. See also *Vascular malformation(s).*
Intracranial herniation, 18, *19, 20*
Intracranial infection, perinatal, 132
Intradural extramedullary neoplasm, 175–177, *176*
Intradural extramedullary process(es), 136, 138t, *139*
Intramedullary neoplasm, 173–175, *174*
Intramedullary process(es), 136, 138t
Intraventricular cysticercosis, *32*
Intraventricular hemorrhage (IVH), 15, 79–80, *81, 129*
Ischemia, 67–78
    arterial occlusion in, 67–72. See also *Arterial occlusion.*
    brain death in, 74–75, *76*
    carotid artery atherosclerosis in, 72–74, *73*
    global, 74, *74, 75*
    hypoperfusion in, 74, *74, 75*
    metabolic conditions in, 76–78, *78*
    spinal cord, 179
    venous infarction in, 75–76, *77*
IVH (intraventricular hemorrhage), 15, 79–80, *81, 129*

J

Jefferson burst fracture, 150, *150*

K

Krabbe's disease, 108

L

Langerhans cell histiocytosis, *64,* 65

Leigh disease, 107
Leptomeningeal cyst, 23, 24
Lesion(s), skull, 62–64, 64t, 64–65
Leukodystrophy, 107, 107
Leukoencephalopathy, progressive
    multifocal, 33–34, 34
Leukomalacia, periventricular,
    128–130, 130
Ligamentous injury, detection of,
    157–158
Lipoma(s), of corpus callosum, 115,
    116
  of filum terminale, 140
Lipomyelomeningocele, 140, 140
Lissencephaly, 119
Lobar hemorrhage, 93
Locked facet, 153
Longitudinal ligament, ossification
    of, 165–166, 167
Low back pain, 161
Lumbar fracture, 155–157, 157,
    158
Lumbar herniated nucleus
    pulposus, 163
Lumbar stenosis, 165, 166
Lung carcinoma, metastasis of,
    51–52
Lymphatic metastasis, 52–56
Lymphoma, 46, 48

M

Magnetic resonance angiography
    (MRA), of carotid artery, 73
  of dissecting aneurysm, 88, 88
  of intracranial aneurysm, 87, 87
  of venous infarction, 76
Magnetic resonance imaging (MRI),
    of acoustic schwannoma, 60, 60
  of adrenoleukodystrophy, 107,
    107
  of aqueductal stenosis, 99
  of arachnoid cyst, 118
  of arachnoiditis, 172
  of arterial occlusion, 69–70, 70,
    71
  of arteriovenous malformations,
    89, 90
  of astrocytoma, 40, 41–43, 43
  of basal ganglia, 3
  of border zone infarction, 74
  of brain, aging of, 108, 108
  of brain abscess, 29
  of brain death, 75
  of brainstem, 6
  of butterfly glioma, 42, 42
  of Canavan's disease, 107, 107
  of caudal regression, 141, 143
  of cavernous angioma, 91, 92
  of cavernous sinus aneurysm, 59
  of cephalocele, 112
  of cerebellopontine angle epider-
    moid tumor, 51

Magnetic resonance imaging (MRI)
    (Continued)
  of cerebral venous thrombosis,
    77
  of cervical spine flexion injuries,
    154
  of Chiari malformations, 112,
    113
  of choroid plexus papilloma, 46
  of choroidal fissure cyst, 118
  of coccidioidomycosis meningitis,
    31
  of colloid cyst, 98
  of corpus callosum, 114, 116
  of craniopharyngioma, 57, 58
  of cryptococcal meningitis, 36
  of cysticercosis, 31
  of Dandy-Walker malformation,
    115
  of Dandy-Walker variant, 117
  of diastematomyelia, 142, 143
  of dorsal dermal sinus, 141, 142
  of ependymoma, 45
  of epidural abscess, 170, 172
  of extra-axial empyema, 28
  of germinoma, 53
  of global ischemia, 75
  of hemangioblastoma, 49
  of herniated nucleus pulposus,
    162, 163
  of herpes encephalitis, 30
  of heterotopic gray matter, 119
  of HIV infection, 33
  of holoprosencephaly, 116
  of hydrocephalus, 97
  of internal capsule, 3
  of intracranial aneurysm, 87
  of intracranial hemorrhage, 79,
    82–84, 82–85, 83t
  of intramedullary neoplasm, 174
  of lipomyelomeningocele, 140,
    140
  of lymphoma, 48
  of medulloblastoma, 47
  of meningeal carcinomatosis,
    176
  of meningioma, 50, 54, 55
  of meningitis, 27
  of mesial temporal sclerosis,
    132, 132
  of metastases, 52, 55
  of midbrain, 4
  of multiple sclerosis, of brain,
    104–105, 104–106
    of spinal cord, 179
  of nerve sheath tumors, 176
  of neurofibromatosis, 123–125
  of olivopontocerebellar degenera-
    tion, 109
  of osmotic myelinolysis, 78, 78
  of osteomyelitis, 170
  of pachygyria, 121
  of pituitary microadenoma, 56,
    57

Magnetic resonance imaging (MRI)
    (Continued)
  of pneumococcal meningitis, 26
  of polymicrogyria, 122
  of pons, 5
  of posterior third ventricle mass,
    98
  of postnatal acquired brain disor-
    ders, 130–132, 131
  of postoperative spine, 166, 168
  of progressive multifocal leu-
    koencephalopathy, 34
  of radiation injuries to brain, 61,
    63–64
  of schizencephaly, 120
  of septo-optic dysplasia, 117
  of spine, 135–137, 136, 137,
    138t, 139
    arteriovenous malformation
      in, 178
    degenerative diseases of, 162
    trauma to, 145, 154, 157, 157–
      158, 159
  of spondylitis, 170
  of subdural hematomas, 14, 14
  of syrinx, 181
  of systemic lupus erythemato-
    sus, 109
  of toxoplasmosis, 35
  of tuberculoma, 31
  of tuberculous meningitis, 30
  of tuberous sclerosis, 125, 126
  of venous angioma, 91, 92
  of venous infarction, 75–76, 77
  of ventricles, 5
  techniques of, 6–9, 8t
Magnetic source imaging (MSI), 10
Mastoiditis, brain abscess from,
    27, 29
MCA (middle cerebral artery), 70,
    70–72, 71
  infarction of, 68, 69
Medulloblastoma, 45–46, 47
  of posterior fossa, 100
Mega cisterna magna, 117, 117
Megalencephaly, 119
Meningeal carcinomatosis, 175,
    176
Meninges, infections of, 31–33
  neoplasms of, 49–51, 54, 55
Meningioma, 49–50, 54, 55
  of cerebellopontine angle, 60–63
  of spine, 175
  of tuberculum sellae, 57–60
Meningitis, 25–27, 26–28, 171, 173
  bacterial, 25
  coccidioidomycosis, 29, 31
  cryptococcal, 34, 36
  meningococcal, 25
  pneumococcal, 25, 26
  tuberculous, 28, 30, 171, 173
Mesial temporal sclerosis, 132, 132
Metabolism, in focal brain damage,
    76–78, 78

Metabolism *(Continued)*
    inborn errors of, 107
Metachromatic leukodystrophy,
    107
Metastasis(es), 51–56, *55*
    cerebrospinal fluid, 56
    hematogenous, 51–52, *55*
    lymphatic, 52–56
    radiographic features of, 64t
Methemoglobin signal, in cerebral
    venous thrombosis, 76, *77*
Microadenoma, pituitary, 56–57,
    57
Midbrain, hemorrhage in, 15, *15*
    on cross-sectional imaging, *4*
Middle cerebral artery (MCA), *70*,
    70–72, *71*
    infarction of, 68, *69*
Mitochondrial disorder(s), 107
Movement disorder(s), 108–110
MRA. See *Magnetic resonance
    angiography (MRA).*
MRI. See *Magnetic resonance
    imaging (MRI).*
MS (multiple sclerosis), brain and,
    103–105, *104–106*
    spinal cord and, 179–180, *180*
MSI (magnetic source imaging),
    techniques of, 10
Mucormycosis, in immunocom-
    promised patient, 34
Multiple myeloma, 62, 65
    radiographic features of, 64t
Multiple sclerosis (MS), brain and,
    103–105, *104–106*
    spinal cord and, *179*, 179–180,
    180
Myelinolysis, osmotic, 76–78, *78*
Myelitis, transverse, 180, *180*
Myelography, of herniated nucleus
    pulposus, 162
    of spinal cord, 136
    of spinal trauma, 145
Myeloma, *62*, 65
    radiographic features of, 64t
Myelomeningocele, 138, *139*

N

Near-drowning, global ischemia
    from, *75*
Neck. See also *Cervical* entries.
    pain in, 161
Necrosis, radiation, *61*, 63–64
Neoplasm(s), brain, 39–65. See
    also *Brain, neoplasms of.*
    intracranial, hemorrhage and,
    94, *94*
    perinatal, 132
    intramedullary compartment,
    136, 138t
    skull, *62–64*, 64t, 64–65
    spinal, 173–177, *174, 176, 177*

Nerve root tumor, *139*
Nerve sheath tumor, 175, *176*
Neural placode, 138
Neural tube defect, 138–140, *139*
Neuritis, optic, 103, *104*
Neurocutaneous syndrome(s),
    120–127
    neurofibromatosis as, 120–124,
        121t, *123–125*
    Sturge-Weber syndrome as, 127,
        128
    tuberous sclerosis as, 124, *125*,
        126
    von Hippel-Lindau syndrome as,
        127
Neurocysticercosis, 30–31, *32*, 32t,
    33
Neurodegenerative disease(s). See
    Degenerative disease(s).
Neuroectodermal tumor, primitive,
    45–46
    of posterior fossa, 100
Neurofibroma, extramedullary
    intradural, 136, 138t
Neurofibromatosis (NF), 120–124,
    121t, *123–125*
Neurofibromatosis-1 (NF-1), 120,
    123
    astrocytoma in, *43*
    diagnostic criteria for, 121t
Neurofibromatosis-2 (NF-2),
    121–122
    cranial findings in, *124*
    diagnostic criteria for, 121t
    spinal tumors in, *125*
Neuroma, 60, *60*
Neuronal migration disorder(s),
    117–119, *119–122*
Neuronal-origin tumor, 48, *50*
Neurosyphilis, 31
Neurulation, 137
NF (neurofibromatosis), 120–124,
    121t, *123–125*
NF-1 (neurofibromatosis-1), 120,
    123
    astrocytoma in, *43*
    diagnostic criteria for, 121t
NF-2 (neurofibromatosis-2),
    121–122
    cranial findings in, *124*
    diagnostic criteria for, 121t
    spinal tumors in, *125*
Non–glial-cell tumor(s), 45–49
    germ-cell tumors in, 48–49, *51–
    53*, 64t
    hemangioblastoma in, 46–48, *49*
    lymphoma in, 46, *48*
    medulloblastoma in, 45–46, *47*
    neuronal-origin tumors in, 48,
    50
    primitive neuroectodermal tu-
    mor in, 45–46
Normal pressure hydrocephalus
    (NPH), 95–96, *97*

Notochord, split, *142*, 143
NPH (normal pressure
    hydrocephalus), 95–96, *97*
Nuclear medicine, in brain death,
    75, *76*
    techniques of, 9–10
Nucleus pulposus, herniation of,
    137, 162–164, *163–165*
    MRI evaluation of, 157

O

Occlusion, arterial, 67–72. See also
    Arterial occlusion.
Odontoid process, fracture
    through, 151, *151*
Oligodendroglioma, 43–45, *45*
Olivopontocerebellar degeneration
    (OPCD), *109*, 110
Optic glioma, 57
Optic neuritis, in multiple
    sclerosis, 103, *104*
Osmotic myelinolysis, 76–78, *78*
Ossification, of posterior
    longitudinal ligament (OPLL),
    165–166, *167*
Osteitis deformans, *63*, 64t, 65
Osteomyelitis, 169, *170*
    radiographic features of, 64t
Osteoporosis circumscripta, in
    Paget disease, *63*, 64t
Otitis, brain abscess from, 27, *29*

P

Pachygyria, 119, *120, 121*
Paget disease, *63*, 64t, 65
Pain, low back, 161
    neck, 161
Papilloma, choroid plexus, *46*
Parasitic brain infection, 29–31,
    32, 32t, *33*
Parenchymal cysticercosis, *32*
Parenchymal hemorrhage, 80, *81*,
    127–128, *130*
Parinaud's syndrome, 99
Pediatric neuroradiology, 111–133
    considerations in, 111
    in congenital brain malforma-
        tions, 111–119. See also
        Brain.
    in craniosynostosis, 132–133,
        133
    in neurocutaneous syndromes,
        120–127. See also *Neurocu-
        taneous syndrome(s).*
    in perinatal problems, 127t,
        127–130, *129, 130*
    in postnatal acquired disorders,
        130–132, *131, 132*
Pelizaeus-Merzbacher disease, 108

Penetrating brain injury, 15–16, *16*
Perched facet, 153
Perinatal infection(s), 35–37, *36*, 37t
Perinatal neuroradiology, 127t, 127–130, *129*, *130*
Periventricular leukomalacia, 128–130, *130*
PET (positron emission tomography), 10
Phakomatoses, 120
Pial arteriovenous malformation, 88–89, *90*
PICA (posterior inferior cerebellar artery), *71*, 72
Pillar fracture, 153
Pineal region, in aqueductal obstruction, 97–99, *99*, 99t
Pituitary adenoma, *56*, 56–57, *57*
Pituitary apoplexy, 57
Pituitary microadenoma, 56–57, *57*
PML (progressive multifocal leukoencephalopathy), 33–34, *34*
PNET (primitive neuroectodermal tumor), 45–46
of posterior fossa, 100
Pneumococcal meningitis, 25, *26*
Polymicrogyria, 119, *122*
Pons, on cross-sectional imaging, *5*
Positron emission tomography (PET), 10
Posterior cerebral artery (PCA), *71*, 72
Posterior fossa mass, in hydrocephalus, 99–100, 100t
Posterior inferior cerebellar artery (PICA), *71*, 72
Posterior longitudinal ligament, ossification of, 165–166, *167*
Postnatal acquired disorder(s), 130–132, *131*, *132*
Postoperative spine, imaging of, 166, *168*
Premature disjunction, 140, *140*
Premature infant, evaluation of, 127t, 127–130, *129*, *130*
Primitive neuroectodermal tumor (PNET), 45–46
of posterior fossa, 100
Progressive multifocal leukoencephalopathy (PML), 33–34, *34*
Proton(s), in MRI, 6–7
Proton-density image(s), 7
Pyogenic abscess, 27t, 27–28, *29*

R

RA (rheumatoid arthritis), 171–173, *174*
Radiation injury, to brain, *61*, 63–64

Radiculopathy, 161
Radiofrequency (RF) pulse, in MRI, 6
Radiography, in degenerative spine diseases, 161–162, *162*
in spinal trauma, 145
of skull lesions, *62–64*, 64t, 64–65
Radionuclide scan, of brain death, *76*
Rathke's cleft cyst(s), 57
Repetition time (TR), 7
Reversible changes, of vascular origin, *109*, 110
Rheumatoid arthritis (RA), 171–173, *174*
Ring-enhancing mass(es), in multiple sclerosis, 105
of brain, 39, 40t
Rotational injury(ies), of cervical spine, 153, *156*
Rubella, congenital, *36*, 37

S

Saccular aneurysm, *81*, 86
Sacrococcygeal teratoma, 143
Sacrum, in caudal regression, *141*, 142
Safety, in CT, 2
in MRI, 9
Sagittal thrombosis, 75, *77*
SAH (subarachnoid hemorrhage), *12*, 15, *15*, 79, *81*
Hunt and Hess grading system of, 86t
with intracranial aneurysms, 85–86
Schizencephaly, 119, *120*
Schwannoma, acoustic, 60, *60*
Sclerosis, hippocampal, 132, *132*
mesial temporal, 132, *132*
multiple, brain and, 103–105, *104–106*
spinal cord and, 179–180, *180*
tuberous, 124, *125*, *126*
Scoliosis, in neurofibromatosis, *123*
SE (spin-echo) sequence, 7
Sellar region mass, *56–59*, 56–60, 60t
Septo-optic dysplasia, 115–116, *117*
Shaken baby syndrome, 130
Shearing brain injury, 16–18, *18*
Shingling, of facet joints, 153
Shock wave injury, 15–16, *16*
Shunt(s), in hydrocephalus, 101, *101*
Sinus, dorsal dermal, 140–142, *141*
Sinus thrombosis, dural, 75–76, *77*
Skull, fractures of, *17*, 18–24, *21*, *22*
CSF leaks in, 20–21

Skull *(Continued)*
depressed, 16, *17*
growing, 21–24, *23*
temporal bone, 21, *23*
lesions of, *62–64*, 64t, 64–65
multiple myeloma of, *62*, 65
Paget disease of, *63*, 65
trauma to. See *Cranial trauma.*
SLE (systemic lupus erythematosus), *109*, 110
Sonography. See *Ultrasound.*
Spetzler grading system, for arteriovenous malformations, 89t
Spinal cord, demyelinating disease of, *179*, 179–180, *180*
ischemia of, 179
MRI evaluation of, 157
tethered, *139*, 142
Spine, congenital disorder(s) of, 137–143
abnormal canalization in, *139*, *141*, 142–143
failure of disjunction in, 140–142, *141*
open neural tube defects as, 138–140, *139*
overview of, 137–138
premature disjunction in, 140, *140*
split notochord syndromes as, *142*, 143
degenerative diseases of, 161–167
clinical features of, 161
clinical management of, 166–167
disc protrusion and herniation in, 162–164, *163–165*
MRI in, 162
postoperative imaging in, 166, *168*
radiography in, 161–162, *162*
stenosis in, 164–166, *166*, *167*
formation of, 137–138
imaging of, 135–137, *136*, *137*, 138t, *139*
infection(s) of, 167–173
arachnoiditis as, 171, *172*
arthritis as, 171–173, *174*
epidural abscess as, 169–171, *172*
meningitis as, 171, *173*
vertebral and intervertebral, 167–169, *169–171*
neoplasms of, 173–177, *174*, *176*, *177*
stenosis of, 164–166, *166*, *167*
trauma to, 145–159
cervical, 146–155. See also *Cervical trauma.*
complications of, 158
MRI in, *154*, *157*, 157–158, *159*

Spine *(Continued)*
    thoracic and lumbar, 155–157, *157, 158*
    vascular diseases of, 177–179, *178*
Spin-echo (SE) sequence, 7
Spinous process(es), avulsion of, 153, *155*
Split notochord syndrome, *142,* 143
Spondylitis, 167, *169, 170*
Spondylolisthesis, 162, *162*
    traumatic, 152, *152*
Spondylolysis, 162, *162*
Staphylococcus aureus spondylitis, 167, *169*
Stenosis, aqueductal, 99, *99*
    spinal, 164–166, *166, 167*
Stroke, 67. See also *Ischemia.*
Sturge-Weber syndrome, 127, *128*
Subarachnoid cysticercosis, *32*
Subarachnoid hemorrhage (SAH), 12, 15, *15,* 79, *81*
    Hunt and Hess grading system of, 86t
    with intracranial aneurysms, 85–86
Subdural effusion, in meningitis, 25–26, *26*
Subdural empyema, in meningitis, 26, *28*
Subdural hematoma, 12, 13–14, *14, 15*
    herniation in, 18, *19, 20*
Subfalcine herniation, 18, *19*
Subluxation, of C6-C7 vertebrae, *146*
Superior sagittal thrombosis, 75, 77
Syphilis, in brain infection, 31
Syringohydromyelia, 180
Syringomyelia, 138t, 180
Syrinx, 180–181, *181*
    Chiari malformations and, 112, *112*
    intramedullary, 136, 138t
Systemic lupus erythematosus (SLE), 109, 110

T

TCD (transcranial Doppler), 9
TE (echo time), 7
Teardrop fracture, flexion, 153
Telangiectasia, capillary, 91–92
Temporal bone fracture, 21, *23*
Temporal sclerosis, mesial, 132, *132*
Tentorial herniation, 18, *20*
Teratoma, 49
    sacrococcygeal, 143
Tethered spinal cord, *139,* 142
Thoracic fracture, 155–157, *157, 158*

Thrombosis, dural sinus, 75–76, 77
Thrombotic infarction, in arterial occlusion, 67–70, *68–71*
    in venous occlusion, 75, 77
Tissue characteristic(s), on CT, 2
    on MRI, 7–8
Tomography, computed. See *Computed tomography (CT).*
    positron emission, 10
T1-weighted MR image(s), 7
    characteristics of, 8t
    of acoustic schwannoma, 60, *60*
    of aqueductal stenosis, *99*
    of arachnoid cyst, *118*
    of astrocytoma, 40, *41, 43, 44*
    of basal ganglia, *3*
    of border zone infarction, *74*
    of brain, abscess of, *29*
        radiation injuries to, *61*
    of brainstem, *6*
    of caudal regression, *141*
    of cavernous angioma, *92*
    of cavernous sinus aneurysm, *59*
    of cephalocele, *112*
    of cerebellopontine angle epidermoid tumor, *51*
    of cerebral venous thrombosis, 77
    of Chiari malformations, *112, 113*
    of choroid plexus papilloma, *46*
    of choroidal fissure cyst, *118*
    of colloid cyst, *98*
    of corpus callosum, *114, 116*
    of cysticercosis, *31*
    of Dandy-Walker malformation, *115*
    of Dandy-Walker variant, *117*
    of diastematomyelia, *142*
    of dorsal dermal sinus, *141*
    of epidural abscess, *170, 172*
    of extra-axial empyema, *28*
    of germinoma, *53*
    of hemangioblastoma, *49*
    of herniated nucleus pulposus, *163*
    of herpes encephalitis, *30*
    of hydrocephalus, *98*
    of internal capsule, *3*
    of intracranial hemorrhage, 82, *82–84*
    of intramedullary neoplasm, *174*
    of lipoma, *116*
    of lipomyelomeningocele, 140, *140*
    of lymphoma, *48*
    of medulloblastoma, *47*
    of meningeal carcinomatosis, *176*
    of meningioma, *54*
    of meningitis, *27*
    of metastases, *55*
    of midbrain, *4*
    of multiple sclerosis, *104*

T1-weighted MR image(s) *(Continued)*
    of myelomeningocele, *139*
    of nerve sheath tumors, *176*
    of neurofibromatosis, *123–125*
    of olivopontocerebellar degeneration, *109*
    of osmotic myelinolysis, 78, *78*
    of osteomyelitis, *170*
    of pituitary microadenoma, *57*
    of pneumococcal meningitis, *26*
    of polymicrogyria, *122*
    of pons, *5*
    of schizencephaly, *120*
    of septo-optic dysplasia, *117*
    of spine, *136*
        postoperative, *168*
    of spondylitis, *170*
    of syrinx, *181*
    of tuberculous meningitis, *30*
    of ventricles, *5*
        mass on, *98*
T2-weighted MR image(s), 7
    characteristics of, 8t
    of acoustic schwannoma, 60, *60*
    of adrenoleukodystrophy, *107*
    of arachnoid cyst, *118*
    of arachnoiditis, *172*
    of arteriovenous malformations, *90*
    of astrocytoma, *42, 43, 44*
    of brain, abscess of, *29*
        multiple sclerosis of, *104, 106*
        of HIV infection, *33*
    of Canavan's disease, *107*
    of cavernous angioma, *92*
    of cavernous sinus aneurysm, *59*
    of cerebellopontine angle epidermoid tumor, *51*
    of cervical spine flexion injuries, *154*
    of choroidal fissure cyst, *118*
    of chronic infarction, *70*
    of corpus callosum, *114*
    of cryptococcal meningitis, *36*
    of CSF leaks, 20–21
    of Dandy-Walker malformation, *115*
    of ependymoma, *45*
    of epidural abscess, *170*
    of germinoma, *53*
    of global ischemia, *75*
    of herniated nucleus pulposus, *163*
    of herpes encephalitis, *30*
    of heterotopic gray matter, *119*
    of holoprosencephaly, *116*
    of intracranial hemorrhage, 82, *82–84*
    of intramedullary neoplasm, *174*
    of lymphoma, *48*
    of meningioma, *54*
    of mesial temporal sclerosis, *132*
    of metastases, *55*

T2-weighted MR image(s)
(Continued)
of nerve sheath tumors, *176*
of neurofibromatosis, *123*
of osmotic myelinolysis, 78, *78*
of osteomyelitis, *170*
of pachygyria, *121*
of polymicrogyria, *122*
of progressive multifocal leukoencephalopathy, *34*
of spinal cord, multiple sclerosis
of, *179*
of spine, *136*
arteriovenous malformation
in, *178*
postoperative, *168*
of spondylitis, *170*
of systemic lupus erythematosus, *109*
of toxoplasmosis, *35*
of tuberous sclerosis, *125*, *126*
of venous infarction, *77*
Toxin(s), in focal brain damage, 76
Toxoplasmosis, in immunocompromised patient, 34, *35*
perinatal, 35
TR (repetition time), 7
Transcranial Doppler (TCD), 9
Transtentorial herniation, 18, *20*
Transverse myelitis, 180, *180*
Trauma, cranial, 11–24. See
Cranial trauma.
postnatal, 130–132, *131*
spinal, 145–159. See also *Spine,
trauma to.*
Tuberculoma, 29, *31*
Tuberculosis, in brain infections,
28–29, *30*, *31*
in immunocompromised patient,
34
Tuberculous meningitis, 28, *30*,
171, *173*
Tuberculum sellae, meningioma of,
57–60
Tuberous sclerosis, 124, *125*, *126*
Tumor(s). See also *Neoplasm(s).*
choroid plexus, 45, *46*

Tumor(s) *(Continued)*
epidermoid, 48, *51*
in failure of disjunction, 140
germ-cell, 48–49, *51–53*, 64t
glial, 40–45. See also *Glioma(s).*
nerve root, *139*
neuronal-origin, 48, *50*
non–glial-cell, 45–49. See also
Non–glial-cell tumor(s).
of von Hippel-Lindau syndrome,
127
primitive neuroectodermal,
45–46
of posterior fossa, 100

U

Ultrasound, 9
of carotid artery, 73
of hydrocephalus, *129*
of intracranial hemorrhage, *129*
techniques of, 9
Uncal herniation, 18, *19*

V

Vascular blush, in meningiomas,
50, *55*
Vascular disease(s), intracranial
hemorrhage in, 79–94. See
also *Intracranial hemorrhage.*
ischemia in, 67–78. See also *Ischemia.*
of spine, 177–179, *178*
Vascular injury, MRI evaluation of,
158
Vascular malformation(s), 88–93
arteriovenous, 88–91, 89t, *90*, *91*
capillary telangiectasia as,
91–92
carotid-cavernous fistula as, 92–
93, *93*
cavernous angioma as, 91, *92*
of spine, 177–179, *178*

Vascular malformation(s)
(Continued)
vein of Galen, 92
venous angioma as, 91, *92*
Vasculitis, 28
Vein of Galen, malformation of, 92
Venous angioma, 91, *92*
Venous infarction, 75–76, 77
Ventricular system, 1–2
in hydrocephalus, 101, *101*
obstruction of, 96–97, 97t, *98*
in multiple sclerosis, 104, *106*
masses of, *98*
on cross-sectional imaging, *5*
Ventriculitis, 26
Vertebral column. See *Spine.*
Vertebral disc, infection of,
167–169, *169–171*
MRI evaluation of, 157
protrusion of, 162–164, *163–165*
Viral infection, of brain, 31–33
Vitreous humor, characteristics of,
on MRI, 8
Volume loss, in arterial occlusion,
70, *72*
von Hippel-Lindau syndrome, 127
von Recklinghausen disease, 120

W

Water, characteristics of, on MRI,
8, 8t
Watershed infarction, 74, *74*
White matter, aging changes of,
108, *108*
characteristics of, on CT, 2
on MRI, 8, 8t
disease of, 105
in Alexander's disease, 107
Window settings, for cranial
trauma, 11, *12*
Wound(s), gunshot, cranial, 15–16,
16